ORGAN
PHYSIOLOGY

STRUCTURE AND FUNCTION OF THE LUNG

With Emphasis on Roentgenology

ROBERT G. FRASER, M.D., F.R.C.P. (C)

Professor of Diagnostic Radiology, McGill University, and
Diagnostic Radiologist-in-Chief, Royal Victoria Hospital, Montreal

J. A. PETER PARÉ, M.D.

Associate Professor of Medicine, McGill University, Joint
Cardiorespiratory Service, Royal Victoria Hospital, Montreal

1971

W. B. SAUNDERS COMPANY • PHILADELPHIA • LONDON • TORONTO

W. B. Saunders Company: West Washington Square
Philadelphia, PA 19105

12 Dyott Street
London, WC1A 1DB

1835 Yonge Street
Toronto 7, Ontario

ORGAN PHYSIOLOGY – Structure and Function of the Lung SBN 0-7216-3858-9

Print No.: 9 8 7 6 5 4 3 2 1

TO OUR WIVES

PREFACE

The undertaking given the authors to prepare a monograph on the structure and function of the normal lung proved relatively simple: since the first chapter of our recent book *Diagnosis of Diseases of the Chest* deals exclusively with structure and function of the normal thorax, little alteration was required to convert it into a separate publication.

Even in the short span of one year since *Diagnosis of Diseases of the Chest* was published in early 1970, knowledge of pulmonary structure and function has been modified and extended; however, new developments have occurred largely in the area of pathologic rather than normal morphology and physiology, and with one exception we have considered it unnecessary to modify the existing text. The exception consists of new material on the bronchographic morphology of the peripheral airways and the roentgenologic appearance of the human pulmonary acinus, material which has been added to the section of the lung unit. In addition, a section dealing with pulmonary function tests has been lifted from Chapter 3 and added to the end of the monograph in order to facilitate understanding of the somewhat complex descriptions of the physiology of respiration. Deletions have been few, consisting mainly of discussions of roentgenologic interpretation which we regarded as noncontributory to a monograph of this nature.

The three major structures of the lung—the lung unit, the airways, and the vascular system—are described in relation to their morphology, their roentgenology, and their function. The remaining constituents of the thorax—the pleura, the lymphatic system, the mediastinum, the diaphragm, and the chest wall—are considered mainly from morphologic and roentgenologic viewpoints, function being discussed only when it is significant. It might be anticipated that a monograph devoted to the structure and function of an organ would contain considerable description of macroscopic and microscopic anatomy but a glance through the pages will reveal abundant illustrations of roentgenograms and but few of gross specimens or histologic sections. Although this lack of emphasis on morphologic anatomy might be justly criticized, we offer no apology for the weight lent roentgenologic description: in practice, the thorough knowledge of thoracic anatomy required for an adequate understanding of diseases of the chest is applied much more frequently in roentgenographic studies than in the dissecting room or necropsy theater.

The bibliography is unchanged from the original work except for the addition of new references.

We think it appropriate that this preface end in the same manner as the preface to *Diagnosis of Diseases of the Chest*: We recognize our fallibility. It is inevitable that some observations in a text of this magnitude will prove erroneous in time or will find disagreement among our knowledgeable readers. This we expect and accept. We sincerely hope that such differences of opinion will be made known to us, so that they may be weighed and, where appropriate, introduced into subsequent editions or revisions. It is only through such interchange of information and opinion that we can hope to establish on a firm basis the knowledge necessary to a full understanding of respiratory disease.

R. G. F.

J. A. P. P.

ACKNOWLEDGMENTS

It is difficult to know how to acknowledge adequately the contributions of others in the production of this monograph. Since its contents have been lifted with only slight modification from the book *Diagnosis of Diseases of the Chest*, it would seem appropriate to mention by name all those who contributed to the production of the much larger work. However, to do so would be tediously repetitious and we will restrict individual acknowledgment to those who contributed most in time and effort to the preparation of the first chapter of the book: Miss Coni Reed and Miss Elizabeth McKee for transcription and typing of manuscript; Miss Catherine Mayhew and Mr. R. S. Fraser for validation of references; and J. Gebhardt Smith for her superb artwork. Dr. W. M. Thurlbeck deserves special mention for his invaluable contributions, specifically for many of the descriptions of morphology which appear throughout the monograph.

Finally, we are indebted to Mr. John L. Dusseau, Vice President and Editor of W. B. Saunders Company, who invited us to prepare the monograph and suggested its general content and format.

THE NORMAL CHEST

THE LUNG UNIT

THE ACINUS AS AN ANATOMIC UNIT

In the bronchial pathway to the periphery of the lungs, the last purely conducting structure is the terminal bronchiole. The portion of the lung distal to the terminal bronchiole is the *acinus*, which comprises respiratory bronchioles, alveolar ducts, alveolar sacs, and alveoli (Figure 1–1). It is in this region that gas exchange takes place. The precise arrangement and exact number of structures that form the acinus are not known, since reconstruction is extremely difficult and tedious. However, it is known that respiratory bronchioles have some alveoli in their walls and that cuboidal epithelium lines the lumen between alveoli. Progressively more alveoli are present in succeeding generations of respiratory bronchioles. Respiratory bronchioles are succeeded by alveolar ducts whose walls are formed by a musculoelastic mesh through which alveoli protrude outward. Alveolar ducts lead to the terminal, blind structures of the respiratory tree—alveolar sacs, which also are lined entirely by alveoli but in which there is no smooth muscle.

A variety of terms has been used for the same structures in the acinus, and the reader is referred to the excellent review by Pump.[8] It seems likely that divisions within the acinus follow a pattern of irregular dichotomy with axial and lateral pathways, as in the conducting system (*see* page 8). Thus, there may be from two to nine generations of respiratory bronchioles. The last respiratory bronchiole gives rise to a complex terminal spray of alveolar ducts and sacs in which dichotomous, trichotomous, or even quadrivial division occurs in irregular fashion. It can be estimated that there are about 400 alveolar ducts and sacs in an acinus and 18 last-order respiratory bronchioles arising from one terminal bronchiole. There are altogether about 14 million alveolar ducts and sacs, which contain the greater portion of the lungs' 300 million alveoli, each of which has a diameter of 250 to 300μ when fully inflated.[9] Alveoli are polygonal and have a continuous lining formed of flattened epithelial cells. In the sharp angles of the alveoli are plumper cells, with oval nuclei and granular cytoplasm. These corner cells, which are known also as type-II or septal cells, have many mitochondria, are metabolically highly active, and contain characteristic osmophilic inclusions which are thought to be the origin of the surface-active material that lines the alveolar surface.[10, 11] The total alveolar surface area is some 40 to 100 sq m, depending upon body size.[12] This area, in which gas transfer takes place, is extremely thin, and Schulz[97] has calculated that the thickness of the pathway from alveolar gas to the plasma layer of

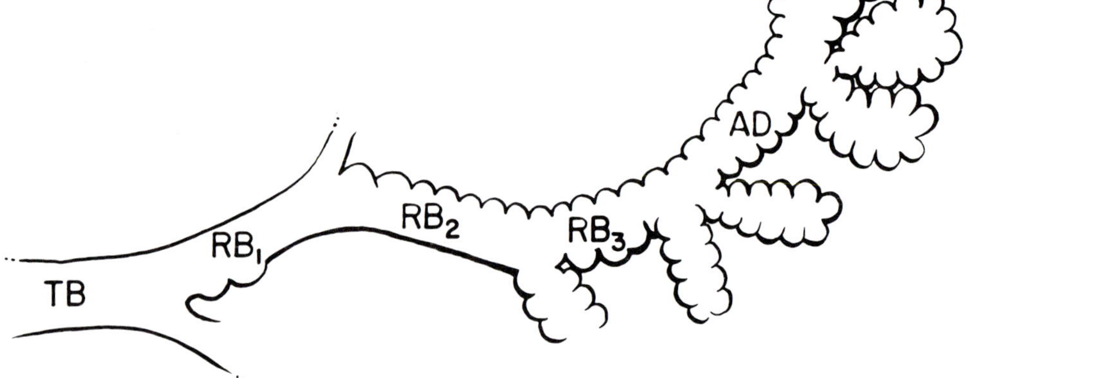

Figure 1–1. **Component Parts of the Acinus.** TB-terminal bronchiole. RB-respiratory bronchiole. AD-alveolar duct. AS-alveolar sac. (Thurlbeck, W. M.: Chronic obstructive lung disease. In: Sommers, S. C. (ed.), *Pathology Annual: Nineteen Sixty-eight.* Appleton-Century-Crofts, 1968, p. 377.)

blood is 0.36 to 2.5μ – a small distance in terms of the diameter of a normal red blood cell.

The Lobule

The lobule is usually defined as the smallest discrete portion of the lung that is surrounded by connective-tissue septa, and corresponds to the "secondary lobule" described by Miller.[4] Since the septa are variable in size and extent, the size of the lobule is variable. It should not be confused with Miller's "primary lobule," which consists of an alveolar duct, its vessels, and the structures arising from them. The secondary lobule rarely is recognizable roentgenographically as a unit of structure; only when edema fluid or other pathologic tissue within the interlobular septa renders these structures visible as septal lines can the volume of lung between two lines be recognized as a secondary lobule. It is obvious that such a limitation negates the usefulness of Miller's definition for purposes of pathologic-roentgenologic correlation.

To overcome this limitation, Reid and Simon[158] proposed an alternate definition, based on a subdivision of peripheral lung structure that is more constant and is recognizable both morphologically and roentgenographically. These authors pointed out that if one follows a bronchial pathway to the periphery of the lung in a well-filled bronchogram (Figure 1–2), a stage is reached at which branching of the parallel-walled pathway occurs every 0.5 to 1.0 cm. After three or four such branchings, an abrupt transition takes place in which the branching patterns occur at 2- to 3-mm intervals. These have been termed the "centimeter" and "millimeter" patterns, respectively. The centimeter pattern of branching represents small bronchi and bronchioles and the millimeter pattern relates to terminal bronchioles. Reid and Simon[158] proposed that the lobule be redefined as the cluster of three to five terminal bronchioles which form the millimeter pattern of branching at the end of a bronchial pathway (either axial or side branch), together with the respiratory tissue it supplies.

In a study of peripheral bronchographic morphology carried out recently in our laboratories, Gamsu and his colleagues[169] injected a special tantalum suspension into selected airways of four excised normal human lungs and correlated the roentgenographic, microradiographic, and histologic appearances of selected areas. They demonstrated a characteristic difference in the appearance of nonrespiratory and respiratory bronchioles, the former possessing a distinct tubular appearance and the latter a rosette or woolly configuration (Figure 1–4*A*). They were unable to demonstrate the simple branching system required to produce the "centimeter-millimeter" pattern and surmised that the pattern described by Reid and Simon[158] must have resulted from incomplete filling of nonrespiratory bronchioles owing to lack of penetration of the radiopaque injection mass beyond terminal bronchioles. It appears that the Gamsu study has established, in convincing fashion, the character of peripheral bronchiolar branching in the human lung; the possibility of identifying terminal bronchioles and of differentiating terminal from respiratory bronchioles on clinical bronchograms should permit considerable extension of our knowledge of the growing list of diseases known to affect the small airways.

Canals of Lambert

The distal portions of the bronchiolar tree, particularly the preterminal bronchioles, contain a number of epithelium-lined tubular communications with surrounding alveoli.[14] The physiologic significance of these structures is not known, but obviously they provide an accessory route for the passage of air directly from the bronchioles into alveoli.

Alveolar Pores

Although these are often called the pores of Kohn, von Hayek[15] attributes their original description to Henle. It is thought that they are present in the lungs of all mammals, though they may be relatively more common in some species. In the human lung, they are openings, or discontinuities, of the alveolar wall, about 10 to 15μ in diameter. The lung distal to an obstructed bronchus or bronchiole may be ventilated via an adjacent airway. This process, known as collateral air drift, is brought about, at least in part, by the pores of Kohn. The lung of the dog has no interlobular

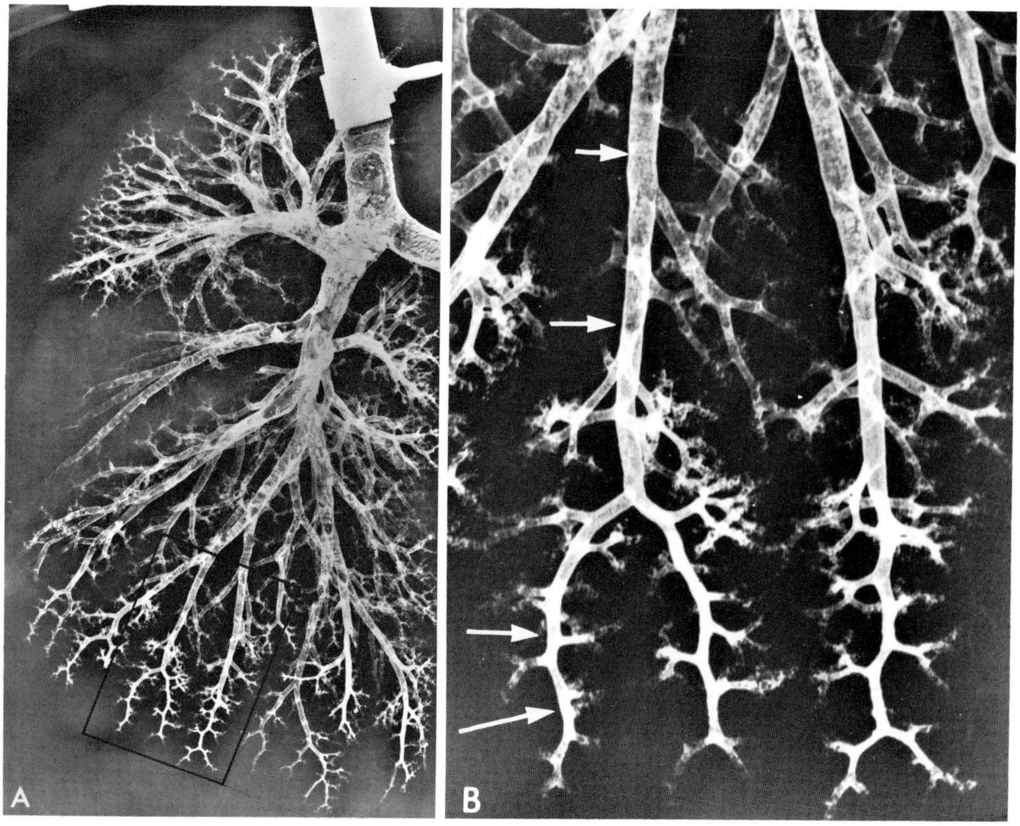

Figure 1–2. **The Pattern of Bronchial and Bronchiolar Branching.** *A*, Roentgenogram of an excised right lung following insufflation of particulate lead into the tracheobronchial tree. *B*, Magnified view of the peripheral airways of the lateral basal segment; upper arrows point to the "centimeter pattern" of branching, lower arrows to the "millimeter pattern." (Roentgenogram through the courtesy of Dr. James Hogg, Department of Pathology, McGill University.)

septa and, therefore, the lobar tissue is continuously interconnected.

Direct Airway Anastomoses

Martin[16] recently showed direct communications between "respiratory bronchioles" in the dog, measuring up to 120μ in diameter, which appeared to cross intersegmental planes. Although termed "respiratory bronchioles" by the author, the figures illustrate communications between what appear to be alveolar ducts. They were found relatively frequently and, because of their large size, may contribute significantly to collateral ventilation.

The Acinus as a Roentgenologic Unit

It is reasonable to assume that since an acinus is a macroscopic structure, it might be visible roentgenologically when completely or partially filled with contrast material or with inflammatory exudate. In 1924 Aschoff[5] suggested that consolidation of a single acinus by tuberculous inflammatory exudate or granulation tissue results in a rosette-like appearance, which he termed the "acino-nodose" lesion (Figure 1–3). Identical shadows were created by Twining[18] in 1931 by overfilling with Lipiodol the bronchial tree of lungs removed at autopsy (Figure 1–4). Neither Aschoff[5] nor Twining[18] proved conclusively that the "acino-nodose" shadow represented a single acinus morphologically and it was not until very recently that the precise roentgenologic nature of the acinus was established. In an extension of their study of peripheral bronchographic morphology to which reference was made previously, Gamsu and his colleagues[170] investigated the feasibility of roentgenographic visualization of individual acini in the human lung. Using a special tantalum suspension, they progressively opacified two segments of normal excised human lungs distal to a wedged catheter, obtaining sequential roentgenographs on fine-grain film until almost total opacification was achieved. By correlating roentgenographic, microradiographic, and histologic appearances, they were able to identify and differentiate terminal and respiratory bronchioles and thus to visualize individual acini: progressive filling of a single acinus initially produced a rosette appearance and eventually a spherical lesion. Measurements of twenty-five acini revealed diameters ranging from 6 to 10 mm, with a mean of 7.4 mm (these figures represent acinar caliber at a volume roughly equivalent to total lung capacity, since the lungs were always roentgenographed at a transpulmonary pressure of 30 cm of water).

In recent years, Ziskind and his associates[19, 20] and Felson[21] have revived a deserved interest in this structure. These authors should be credited with bringing into proper perspective the importance of the recognition of "alveolar-filling" diseases that produce the roentgenographically visible rosette shadows or acinar pattern. In conditions such as pulmonary

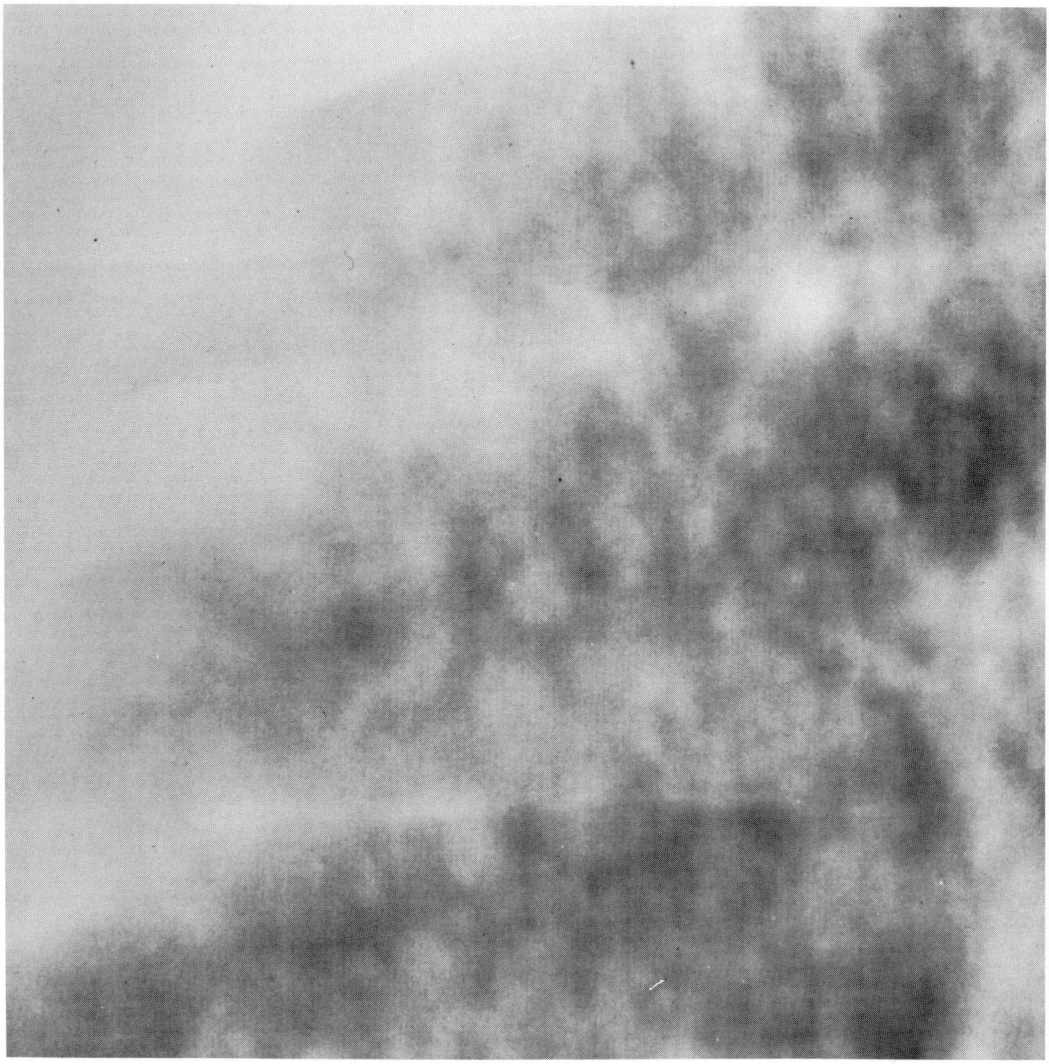

Figure 1–3. **Acinar Shadows.** Magnified view of a tomographic section of the right upper lobe of a patient with bronchogenic spread of tuberculosis from a cavity in the right lower lobe (not illustrated). On the original roentgenogram, individual acinar shadows measured 4 to 5 mm in diameter.

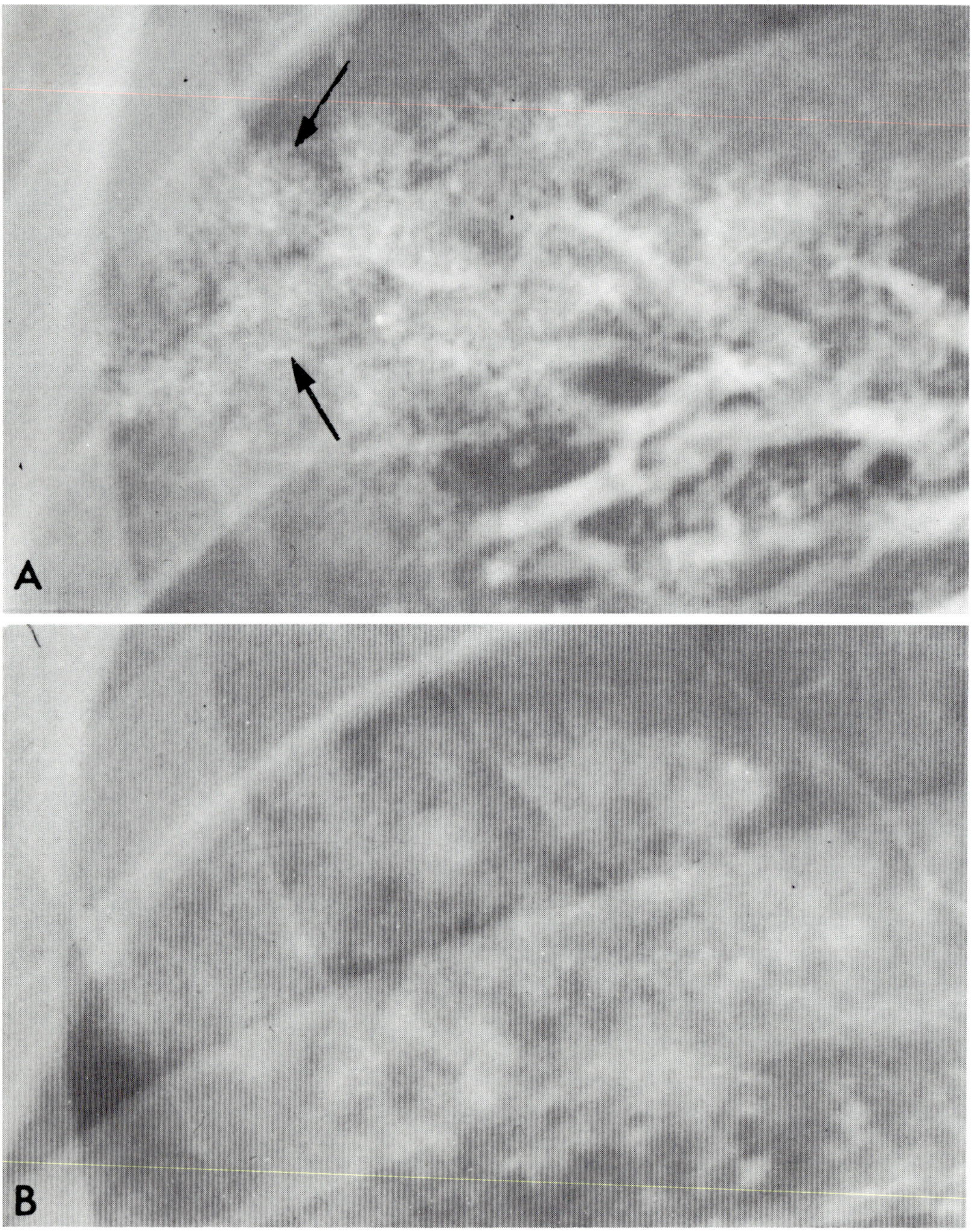

Figure 1–4. **Acinar Shadows.** *A,* Peripheral filling of respiratory bronchioles during bronchography (arrows). *B,* 24 hours later the contrast agent has absorbed but has incited an acute air-space edema resulting in the "rosette" shadows of acinar consolidation.

edema, acute alveolar pneumonia, and idiopathic pulmonary hemorrhage, recognition of this distinctive pattern enables the roentgenologist to narrow the differential diagnosis down to the relatively few diseases capable of consolidating parenchymal air spaces (Figure 1–5).

THE ACINUS AS A FUNCTIONAL UNIT

As defined, the lung unit, which is analogous to the nephron of the kidney, is that portion of the lung parenchyma distal to the terminal bronchiole. This definition is highly acceptable to both anatomists and roentgenologists, but is there evidence that this portion of lung is also a functional unit? Most physiologists describe the alveolus as the unit of the lung. However, in so doing, they do not equate this with the anatomic alveolus but rather with a hypothetical unit which, because of our lack of knowledge of correlation between physiology and anatomy, cannot be defined morphologically. In fact, it would be unrealistic to consider the structural alveolus a physiologic unit. Each alveolus is one of a family of 20 or thereabouts, arising from a common alveolar duct and receiving from a common arteriole capillaries which connect the alveoli with one another.[22, 23] It is

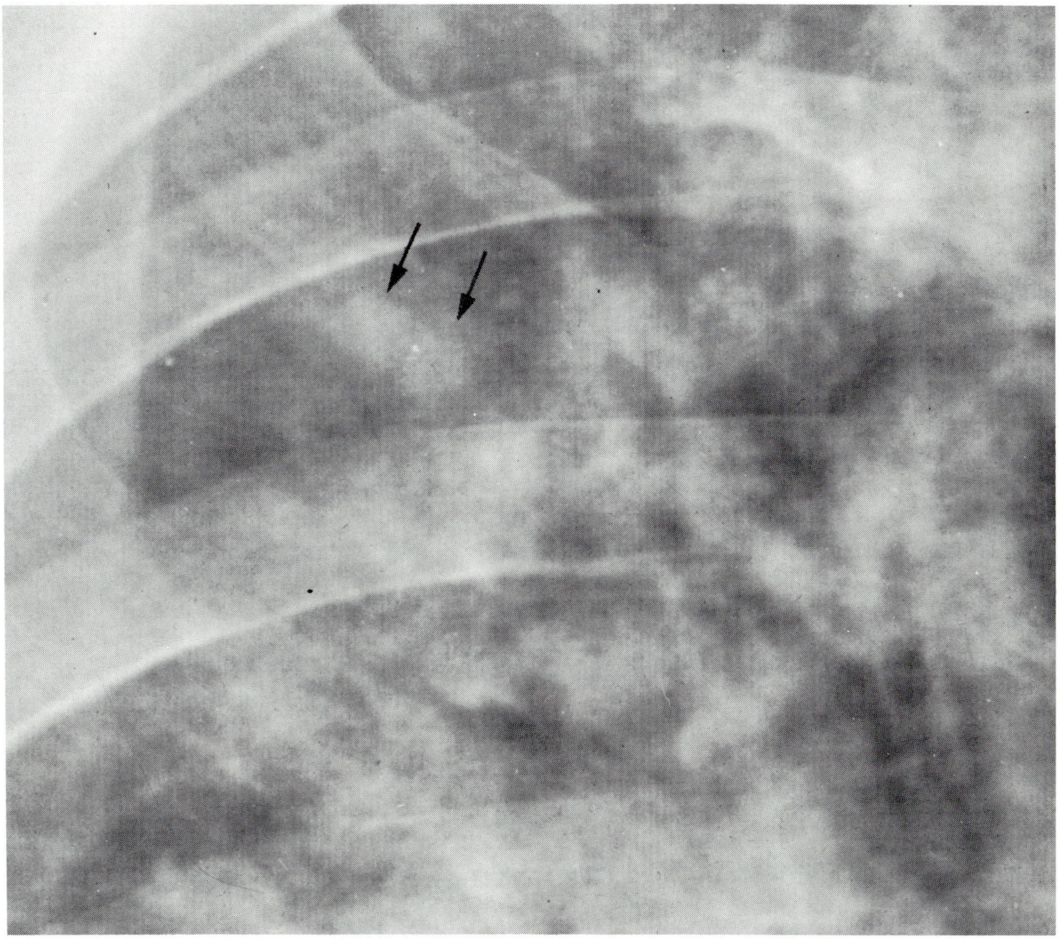

Figure 1–5. **Air-space Consolidation in Acute Pulmonary Edema.** Magnified view (right upper lobe) of the roentgenogram of a patient with diffuse pulmonary edema resulting from aspiration of liquid gastric contents. Air-space consolidation is largely confluent but two relatively discrete acinar shadows can be seen near the center of the field (arrows).

unlikely that, in normal circumstances, the behavior of any one alveolus differs from that of its "siblings." Thus, it seems likely that Miller's primary lobule,[4] comprising the alveolar duct and its ramifications that arise from a third-order respiratory bronchiole, is the smallest portion of lung that can be considered in the concept of a physiologic unit of lung function. Farther up the bronchial tree at the level of the terminal bronchiole, a greater portion of lung is included as a unit of function, since distal to this point there are some 400 alveolar-duct units. Do the 8000 alveoli that make up this acinus behave similarly? This question cannot be answered yet, although accumulating evidence on grounds of both structure and physiology suggest that they do (as will be discussed in relation to ventilation/perfusion ratios). For this reason, and in order to envisage a physiologic counterpart of the morphologic and roentgenologic unit, the basic functioning unit of the lung is taken to be the acinus, *i.e.*, all of that portion of the lung parenchyma distal to the terminal bronchiole.

THE AIRWAYS AND PULMONARY VENTILATION

Morphology

The function of the bronchial tree is to conduct air to the alveolar surface, where gas transfer takes place between respired air and gas dissolved in the blood of the alveolar capillaries. The inspired air should be evenly distributed to the alveolar capillary bed, with minimal resistance to flow. In addition, the bronchi and lungs must be able to protect themselves against noxious external agents, whether these be physical, chemical, or biological. The greater part of the length and the smaller part of the volume of the respiratory tract is concerned only with the conduction of air; this part comprises bronchi and bronchioles, which differ in that there is cartilage in the walls of the former. The remaining part of the tract is the acinus, which is concerned with both conduction and gas exchange, the latter function assuming greater importance distally.

Bronchi and Bronchioles

Bronchial and bronchiolar division generally is dichotomous, but the divisions from the parent bronchus often are unequal and the distance between bronchial divisions quite variable, producing a pattern of irregular branching. When the two branches are of approximately equal size, their cross-sectional area is about 20 per cent greater than that of the parent branch and their angles of branching are equal. When they are of unequal size the smaller branch deviates more from the line of direct continuation of the parent bronchus. When the distance from the main bronchus to the periphery of the lung is small, as in the lung substance at the hilum, small branches from the parent bronchus form a spiral; these are called lateral pathways. When the distance is great, the branches are of about equal size, producing approximately linear (axial) pathways. The number of bronchi in the pathways varies considerably, depending upon the distance from hilum to periphery; thus, there may be as few as six generations of bronchi and bronchioles in a lateral pathway and as many as 15 in an axial one. These extreme variations are illustrated in Table 1–1.

The cartilages of the main-stem bronchi are horseshoe-shaped, as in the trachea (Figure 1–6). In lobar and segmental bronchi they consist of irregularly shaped plates which form much of the wall. As the pathway proceeds distally, the cartilages become progressively smaller and less complete until finally, in bronchi about 1 to 2 mm in diameter, they surround only the origins of the bronchioles arising from them. The bronchial muscle lies between the open ends of the horseshoe-shaped cartilages in the major bronchi, where it is attached to the inner perichondrium about 1 mm from their ends. As the cartilages diminish in size and become irregular, the attachments extend further along the cartilages until, finally, the bronchi are encircled by muscle. In the smaller bronchi and the bronchioles, the muscle bundles form a crisscrossed, spiral, geodesic network.

The epithelium of the bronchi is of pseudostratified ciliated type and contains numerous goblet cells. As the pathway proceeds distally the epithelium becomes progressively thinner, to become single-layered in the bronchioles, and the number of goblet cells decreases. In the terminal bronchioles, the goblet cells and cilia have disappeared and the epithelium has become flattened. The origin of mucus found

Table 1–1. Bronchial and Bronchiolar Division

STRUCTURE	GENERATION FROM TRACHEA	GENERATION FROM SEGMENTAL BRONCHUS	GENERATION FROM TERMINAL BRONCHIOLE	NUMBER	DIAMETER	CROSS-SECTIONAL AREA	
Trachea	0			1	2.5 cm	5 sq cm	Cartilaginous conducting structures
Main bronchi	1			2	11-19 mm	3.2 sq cm	
Lobar bronchi	2/3			5	4.5-13.5 mm	2.7 sq cm	
Segmental bronchi	3/6	0		19	4.5-6.5 mm	3.2 sq cm	
Subsegmental bronchi	4/7	1		38	3-6 mm	6.6 sq cm	
Bronchi		2-6		various	various	various	
Terminal bronchi		3-7		1000	1.0 mm	7.9 sq cm	
Bronchioles		5-14		various	various	various	No cartilage in their walls
Terminal bronchiole		6-15	0	35,000	0.65 mm	116 sq cm	
Respiratory bronchioles			1-8	various	various	various	
Terminal respiratory bronchiole			2-9	630,000	0.45 mm	1000 sq cm	
Alveolar ducts and sacs			4-12	14×10^6	0.40 mm	1.71 sq m	
Alveoli				300×10^6	0.25-0.30 mm	70 sq m (surface area)	

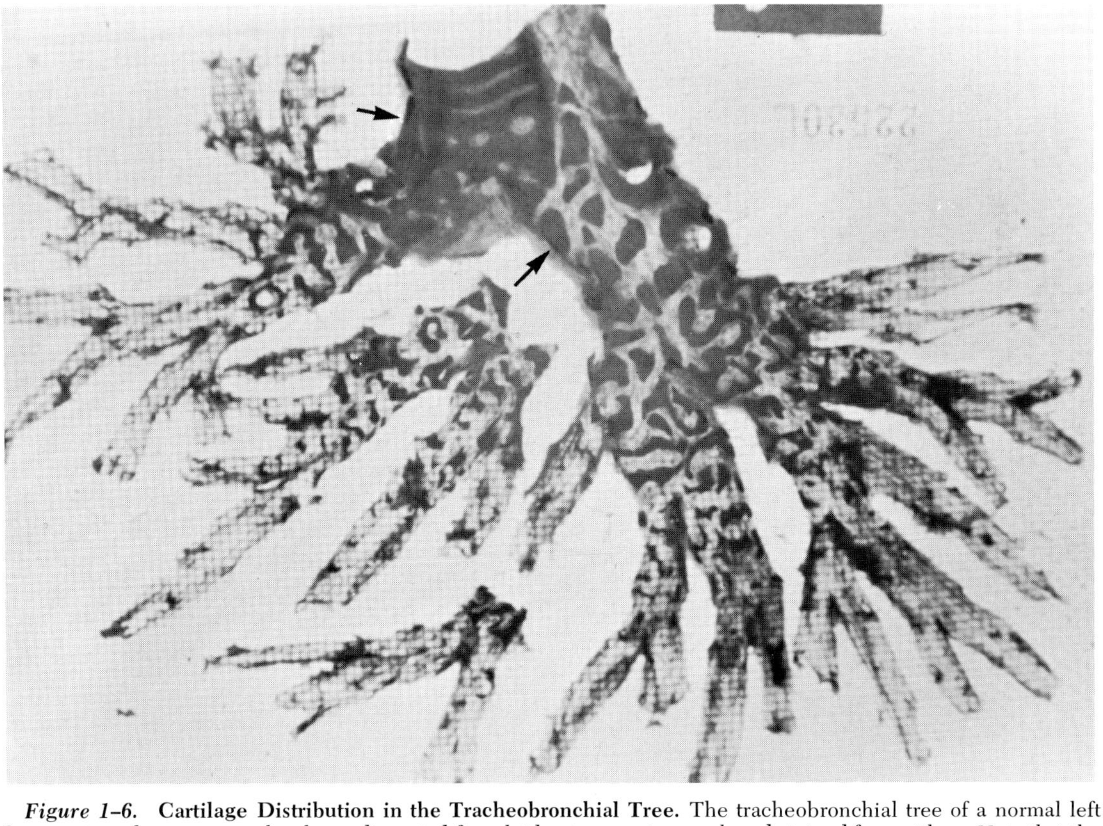

Figure 1–6. **Cartilage Distribution in the Tracheobronchial Tree.** The tracheobronchial tree of a normal left lung removed at necropsy has been dissected free, laid out on a wire mesh and stained for cartilage. *Note* that the horseshoe-shaped cartilages in the trachea (upper arrow) extend for a short distance into the upper-lobe bronchus but that the cartilage in the lower-lobe bronchus (lower arrow) and peripheral bronchi form discrete islands.

in these bronchioles is not known, though it has been shown not to originate from mucous glands of the bronchi; von Hayek[24] believes it to be a special secretion of cells that bulge into the lumen of the bronchiole (Clara cells[25]). There is some evidence that the excessive mucous secretion rich in eosinophils that occurs in asthma may be the product of these cells.

Underneath the epithelium is the basement membrane, and deep to this is the membrana propria, which is composed of loose fibrous tissue with a rich capillary network. The bronchial mucous glands belong to the membrana propria but frequently extend externally to the cartilage or muscle wall. The glands are mixed tubuloacinar in type and usually are termed mixed serous and mucous glands; in fact, the gland acini are more appropriately designated distended or nondistended (by mucus).[26] It seems likely that cyclic production of mucus converts one to the other, since mucopolysaccharides are present in "serous" acini also. Mucous glands extend to the small bronchi, roughly paralleling the distribution of cartilage. The volume of bronchial mucous glands is much greater than that of goblet cells, and it is likely that bronchial glands secrete most of the mucus contained in the tracheobronchial tree. Bands of longitudinal elastic fibers form dense bundles in the membrana propria, causing a ridging of the bronchi that becomes less conspicuous distally. These longitudinal elastic fibers connect with circularly arranged elastic fibers that are in relation to the muscular layer and, in the small bronchioles, through the circular elastic fibers to the surrounding alveolar and septal elastic tissue, thus forming a continuum through the lungs. It is believed that this radial tethering mechanism plays a major part in maintaining patency of the bronchioles. The peribronchial connective tissue surrounds the bronchi to the point where the bronchiolar walls become continuous with lung parenchyma. It is continuous with the periarterial connective tissue and, near the hilum, with the perivenous connective tissue. At the hilum and at the periphery of lobules there is continuity between the interlobular (septal) connective tissue and the subpleural connective tissue.

The Limiting Membrane

The true lung parenchyma (alveoli) is sharply delineated from surrounding connective tissue by a limiting membrane which is composed of dense elastic tissue and collagen and which merges into the elastic fibers of alveolar walls.[15] The membrane forms a boundary between alveolar parenchyma and the loose connective tissue of the bronchovascular tree, the interlobar septa, and the pleura; the loose connective tissue at the latter site constitutes the subpleural connective tissue or vascular layer of the pleura (*see* page 59). Blood vessels, nerves, and lymphatics lie in these compartments of loose connective tissue, which together form the interstitial space. Pressure may be more negative in this space than in the pleural cavity, and air and fluid readily accumulate there.

Roentgenology

It is of obvious importance for physicians interested in diseases of the chest to be familiar with the terminology and general spatial distribution of the bronchi and of the bronchopulmonary segments they supply. However, the number of variations from the norm of subdivision of the bronchial tree precludes detailed consideration of the subject in this book.* In addition, we feel that a thorough understanding of pulmonary disease requires more a familiarity with the anatomy of bronchopulmonary segments, the zones or regions of the lung supplied by the segmental bronchi, than with detailed knowledge of bronchial branching, since the former is only roughly dependent upon the latter.

Knowledge of segmental bronchial terminology and the mode of bronchial branching is important for two main reasons. (1) Surgical resection for localized disease, notably bronchiectasis, often can be limited to segments: it is desirable to remove no more pulmonary tissue than is necessary

*Bronchial anatomy has been described in detail in several articles by Boyden, Scannell, and their associates,[27-33] and in the monographs by Boyden[34] and by Bloomer and associates,[35] and the interested reader is directed to those sources for detailed information.

for cure. (2) The bronchoscopist may need assistance from bronchographic findings to determine which segment is affected; intrabronchial conditions such as a small peripheral bronchogenic carcinoma or a small foreign body may be situated sufficiently far in the periphery of the lung as to remain undetected during standard bronchoscopic examination.

In this section, therefore, it will suffice to present a standard nomenclature of bronchopulmonary anatomy and to describe the prevailing pattern of segmental bronchial branching; minor variations in the pattern that occur fairly frequently will be indicated.

In 1943 Jackson and Huber[36] published a nomenclature of the bronchial segments which was widely adopted and which remains the generally accepted terminology in North America (*see* Table 1–2). The terminologies recommended by the Thoracic Society of Great Britain in 1949 introduced minor variations of the Jackson and Huber nomenclature.[37] In 1955 Boyden[34] introduced a numerical system for identification of bronchial segments which also is widely used. Although these three variations are included in the table, the Jackson-Huber nomenclature is used exclusively throughout this book.

It is interesting that no official nomenclature exists for the major bronchi interposed between the trachea and the segmental bronchi of the five pulmonary lobes. Through common usage, the designation "main bronchi" is applied to the major bronchi arising from the bifurcation of the trachea down to the origin of the upper-lobe bronchus on each side, and "intermediate bronchus" to the segment between the right upper-lobe bronchus and the origins of the right middle- and lower-lobe bronchi.

The Trachea and Main Bronchi

The trachea is, to all intents and purposes, a midline structure; a slight deviation to the right after entering the thorax is a normal finding and should not be misinterpreted

Table 1–2. *Nomenclature of Bronchopulmonary Anatomy**

JACKSON-HUBER	BOYDEN	BROCK	THORACIC SOCIETY OF GREAT BRITAIN
UPPER LOBE			
Apical	B^{1}	Apical	Apical
Anterior	B^{2}	Pectoral	Anterior
Posterior	B^{3}	Subapical	Posterior
RIGHT MIDDLE LOBE			
Lateral	B^{4}	Lateral	Lateral
Medial	B^{5}	Medial	Medial
RIGHT LOWER LOBE			
Superior	B^{6}	Apical	Apical
Medial Basal	B^{7}	Cardiac	Medial basal
Anterior Basal	B^{8}	Anterior basal	Anterior basal
Lateral Basal	B^{9}	Middle basal	Lateral basal
Posterior Basal	B^{10}	Posterior basal	Posterior basal
LEFT UPPER LOBE			
Upper Division			Upper division
Apical-Posterior	$B^{1\&3}$	Apical and subapical	Apicoposterior or apical and posterior
Anterior	B^{2}	Pectoral	Anterior
Lower (Lingular) Division			Lingular (lower) division
Superior Lingular	B^{4}	Superior lingular	Superior lingular
Inferior Lingular	B^{5}	Inferior lingular	Inferior lingular
LEFT LOWER LOBE			
Superior	B^{6}	Apical	Apical
Anteromedial	$B^{7\&8}$	Anterior	Anterior basal
Lateral Basal	B^{9}	Middle basal	Lateral basal
Posterior Basal	B^{10}	Posterior basal	Posterior basal

*Modified slightly from Hinshaw, H. C., and Garland, L. H.: Diseases of the Chest, W. B. Saunders Co., Philadelphia, 1963, with permission of the authors and publisher.

as evidence of displacement (Figure 1–7*A*). Its walls are parallel except on the left side just above the bifurcation, where a smooth indentation caused by aortic impression commonly exists; rarely a smaller indentation is present at the tracheobronchial angle on the right side, due to the azygos vein. Bronchographically, the trachea, main bronchi, and intermediate bronchus have a smoothly serrated contour, created by the indentations of the horseshoe-shaped cartilage rings positioned at regular intervals along these structures. A deficiency of the cartilage rings (the open end of the horseshoe) is closed by a pliable membranous sheath which produces a flat contour posteriorly.

The trachea divides into the two major bronchi at the carina. The angle of bifurcation is variable and is most acute in asthenic subjects. The course of the right main bronchus distally is more direct than the left—a fact of considerable importance in relation to aspiration; Weingärtner, quoted by von Hayek,[15] has stated that the carinal angle may vary from 50 to 100 degrees, the angles which the right and left major bronchi make with the median plane in these two extremes being 20°/30° to 45°/55°. The transverse diameter of the right main bronchus at total lung capacity is greater than that of the left (15.3 mm, compared with 13.0 mm[38]), although its length before the origin of the upper-lobe bronchus as measured at necropsy is shorter (average, 2.2 cm, compared with 5 cm on the left[39,40]).

The air column of the trachea, both major bronchi and the intermediate bronchus should be plainly visible on well-exposed standard roentgenograms of the chest in frontal projection (*see* Figure 1–67, page 92).

The Lobar Bronchial Segments

On this and the following pages, the anatomic distribution of the bronchial segments is described and illustrated. Each segmental bronchus is considered separately, preceded by reproductions of a right bronchogram and corresponding drawings in posteroanterior (Figure 1–7) and lateral (Figure 1–8) projections, and of a left bronchogram similarly depicted (Figures 1–19 and 1–20).

Right Upper Lobe. The bronchus to the right upper lobe arises from the lateral aspect of the main-stem bronchus approximately 3 cm from the carina. The upper-lobe bronchus divides at slightly more than 1 cm from its origin, most commonly, into three branches.[28,30,35] (Figures 1–9 to 1–11). The pattern of branching in the right upper lobe is variable, particularly in relation to the supply of the axillary portion of the lobe, and reference to the aforementioned literature is recommended to those who desire more detailed information on this subject. Of some interest, although of no definite significance, is the relatively infrequent origin of the upper-lobe bronchus or of one of its branches (usually the apical bronchus) from the lateral wall of the trachea (the "tracheal bronchus").

Right Middle Lobe. The intermediate bronchus continues distally for 3 to 4 cm from the take-off of the right upper-lobe bronchus and then bifurcates to become the bronchi to the middle and lower lobes. The middle-lobe bronchus arises from the anterolateral wall of the intermediate bronchus, almost opposite the origin of the superior segmental bronchus of the lower lobe; 1 to 2 cm beyond its origin it bifurcates into lateral and medial segments (Figures 1–12 and 1–13).

Right Lower Lobe. The first segment to originate in the lower lobe, the superior segmental bronchus (Figure 1–14), arises from the posterior aspect of the lower-lobe bronchus immediately beyond its origin; thus, it is almost opposite the take-off of the middle-lobe bronchus. The four basal segments of the lower lobe may be identified with ease roentgenologically by applying a few basic principles of anatomy. Reference to Figures 1–15 to 1–18 will show that in the frontal projection of a well-filled bronchogram, the order of the basal bronchi from the lateral to the medial aspect of the hemithorax is *anterior/lateral/posterior/medial.* As the patient is rotated into 45-degree oblique and lateral projections, the relationship anterior/lateral/posterior is maintained; hence the mnemonic "A.L.P.," which has been employed advantageously by Nelson.[41] As pointed out by him, the relationship of one basal bronchus to another is easily recognized by use of the A.L.P. designation, the medial basal segment being projected between the lateral and posterior segments in the 45-degree oblique projection and between the anterior and lateral segments in the lateral projection.

LEFT UPPER LOBE. The left main bronchus is somewhat longer than the right, measuring approximately 5 cm in length. About 1 cm beyond its origin from the anterolateral aspect of the main bronchus, the bronchus to the left upper lobe either bifurcates or trifurcates, usually the former. In the bifurcation pattern, the upper division almost immediately divides again into two segmental branches, the apical posterior and anterior (Figures 1–21 and 1–22). The lower division is the lingular bronchus, which is roughly analogous to the middle-lobe bronchus of the right lung. When trifurcation of the left upper-lobe bronchus occurs, the apical posterior, anterior, and lingular bronchi originate simultaneously. As in the right upper lobe, the bronchial supply to regions of the left upper lobe is variable.[27, 29]

The lingular bronchus extends antero-inferiorly for 2 to 3 cm before bifurcating into superior and inferior divisions (Figures 1–23 and 1–24).

LEFT LOWER LOBE. With one exception, the divisions of the left lower-lobe bronchus are identical in name and anatomic distribution to those of the right lower lobe (Figures 1–25 to 1–28). The exception lies in the absence of a separate medial basal bronchus, the anterior and medial portions of the lobe being supplied by a single anteromedial bronchus—although Boyden[34] prefers to designate two separate basal bronchi, the anterior and medial, as on the right side. The mnemonic A.L.P. applies as well to the left lower lobe as to the right for identification of the order of basilar bronchi and their relationship to one another in frontal, oblique, and lateral projections.

Tracheobronchial Anomalies

It may be difficult to decide whether deviation from the prevailing pattern of bronchial branching should be classified as truly anomalous or as a minor variation in the norm. Obviously, any such deviation may be important to the surgeon in determining his approach to pulmonary resection. For example, the tracheal bronchus, and "mirror-image" bronchial trees (bronchial isomerism), may be associated with cardiovascular anomalies or situs inversus, and their presence should be brought to the attention of the surgeon when operative intervention is planned. Many bronchial anomalies, *e.g.*, bronchial atresia or agenesis, produce alteration in lung density.

FUNCTION

The purpose of respiration is to supply oxygen for the metabolic needs of cells and to remove carbon dioxide, one of the waste products of cellular metabolism. In the unicellular organism this is accomplished simply by diffusion of these gases across the cell membrane. In man, although the basic purpose is the same, a complex mechanism is required to accomplish it. To bring oxygen from the atmosphere into contact with the cell membrane requires not only passage of the air down a long system of branching tubes, but also an additional means of transport to convey oxygen to even the most distant cells. This process utilizes two areas of diffusion, one in which oxygen is taken up by blood in pulmonary capillaries, and the other where oxygen arrives at the tissue membrane. The elimination of carbon dioxide is accomplished by the same procedure, but in reverse: diffusion from tissues into blood, and then conveyance to lung capillaries, where the gas diffuses from liquid to gas phase and moves up the tubular conducting system and is exhaled.

Normal lung function requires the provision at the alveoli of sufficient oxygen to satisfy the demands of the tissues and sufficient movement of gas in the tracheobronchial tree to eliminate carbon dioxide brought to the alveoli. The needs of the tissues for oxygen—and consequently, the quantity of carbon dioxide eliminated—vary considerably, owing mainly to muscle activity. At rest, the oxygen requirement may be 200 to 250 ml/min, whereas during maximal exercise it may increase to 20 times this amount. To satisfy this variation in oxygen need in normal circumstances, a similar increase in volume of ventilation is necessary. This is accomplished by stimuli from various sources, the origin depending upon the circumstances of the need: Oxygen lack, carbon dioxide excess in the

(Text continued on page 30)

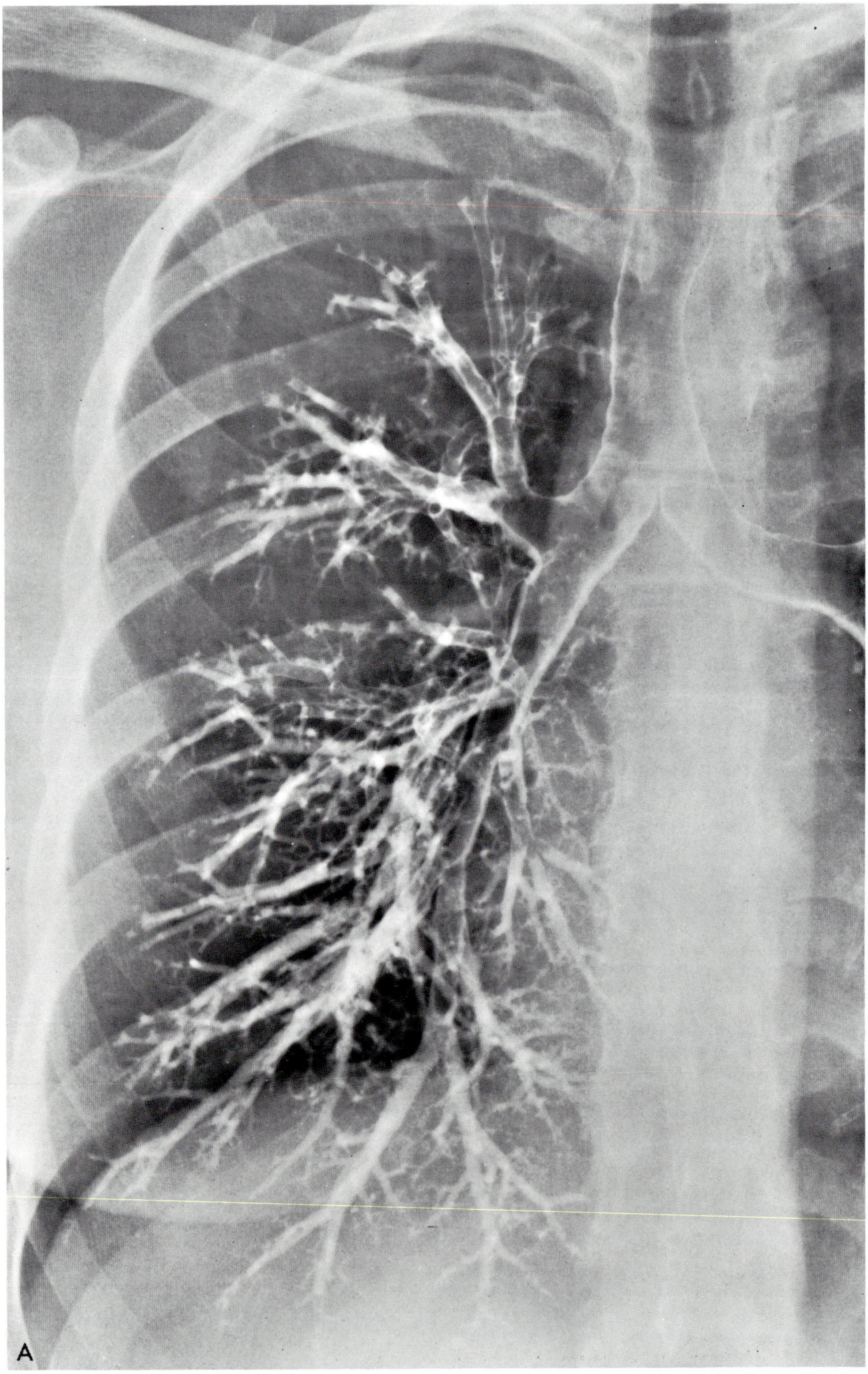

Figure 1–7. **Right Bronchial Tree (Frontal Projection).** *A*, Normal bronchogram of a 39-year-old woman.

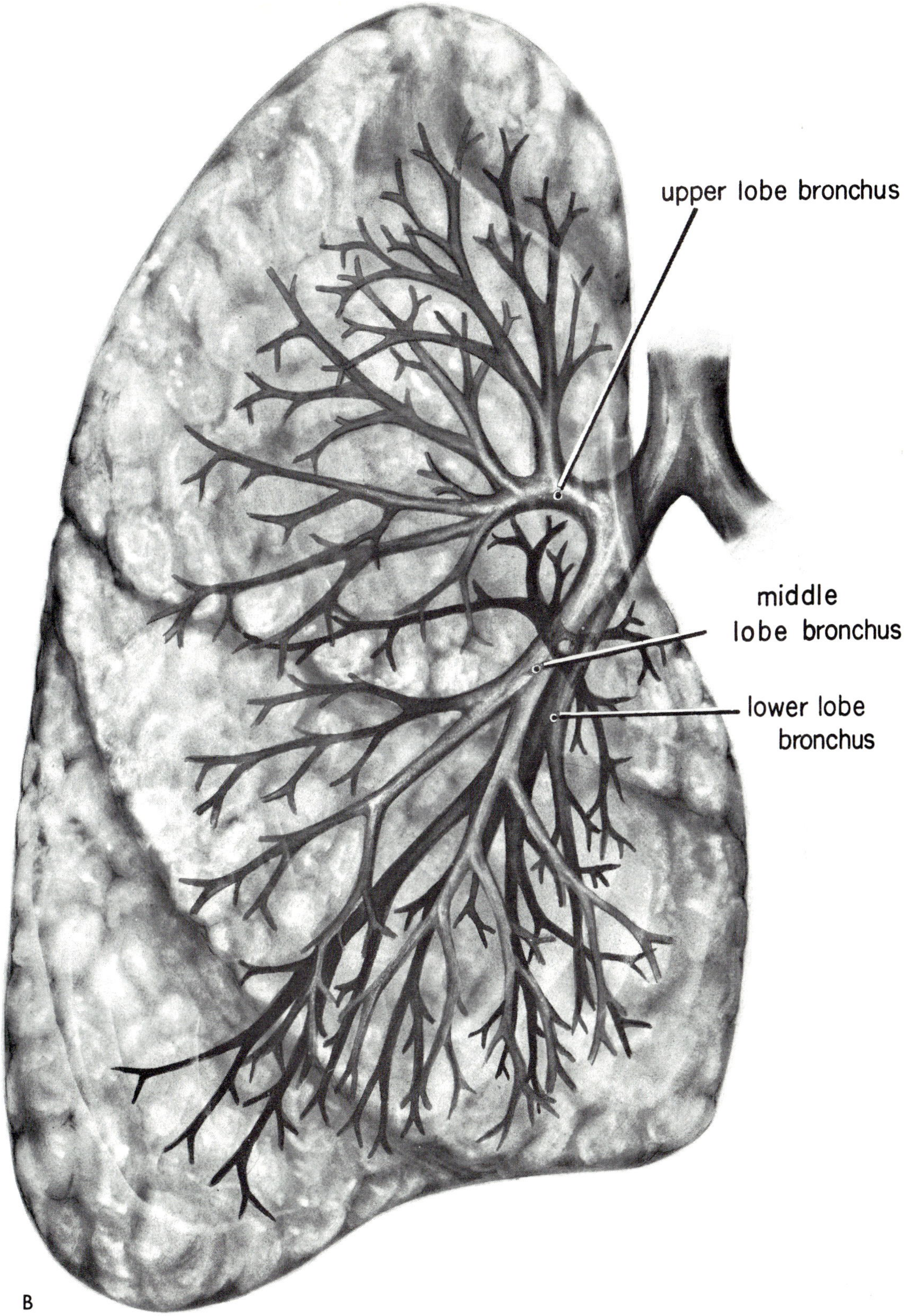

Figure 1-7. *Continued. B,* Semidiagrammatic drawing. *See* Figures 1-8 to 1-18, inclusive, for anatomic distribution of individual segmental bronchi.

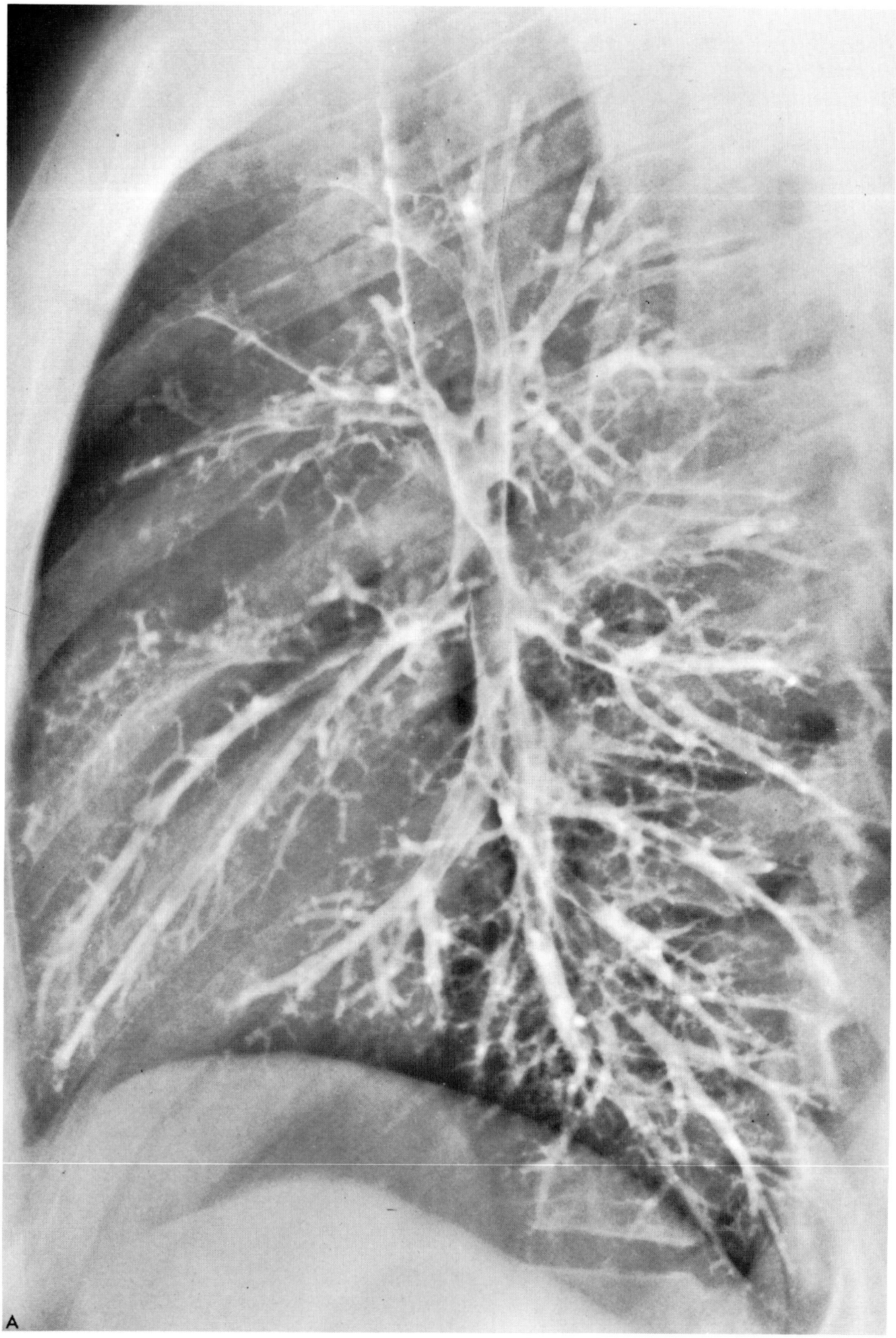

Figure 1–8. **Right Bronchial Tree (Lateral Projection).** *A*, Normal bronchogram of a 39-year-old woman.

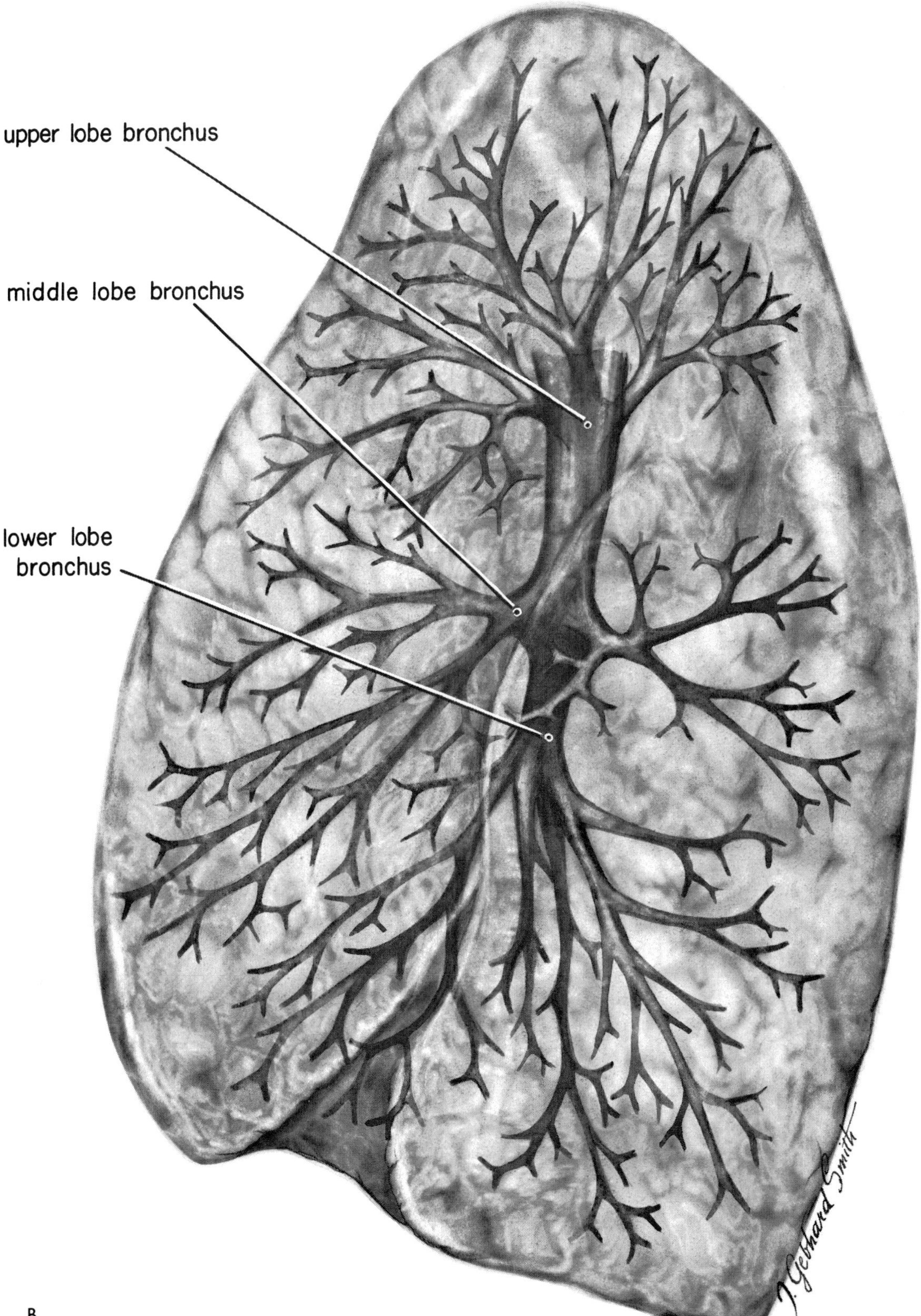

Figure 1–8. Continued. B, Semidiagrammatic drawing. *See* Figures 1–8 to 1–18, inclusive, for anatomic distribution of individual segmental bronchi.

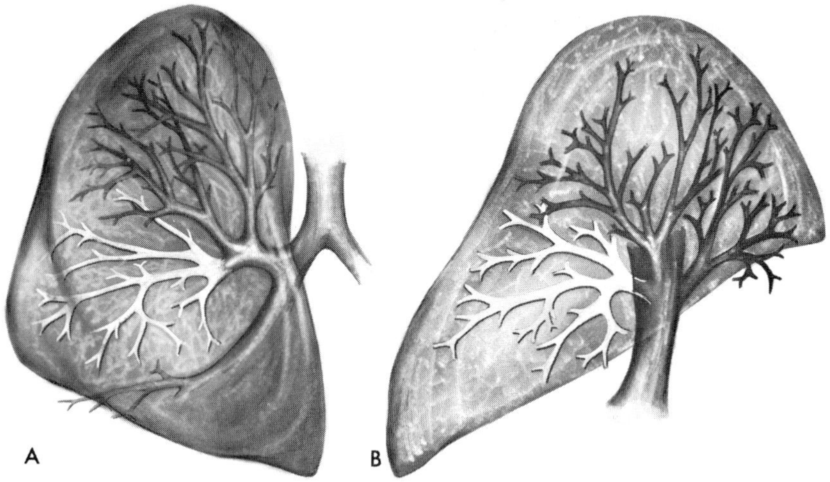

Figure 1–9. **Anterior Segmental Bronchus, Right Upper Lobe.** *A*, Frontal projection; *B*, lateral projection. This segment is directed anteriorly and laterally to supply that portion of the upper lobe contiguous to the minor fissure.

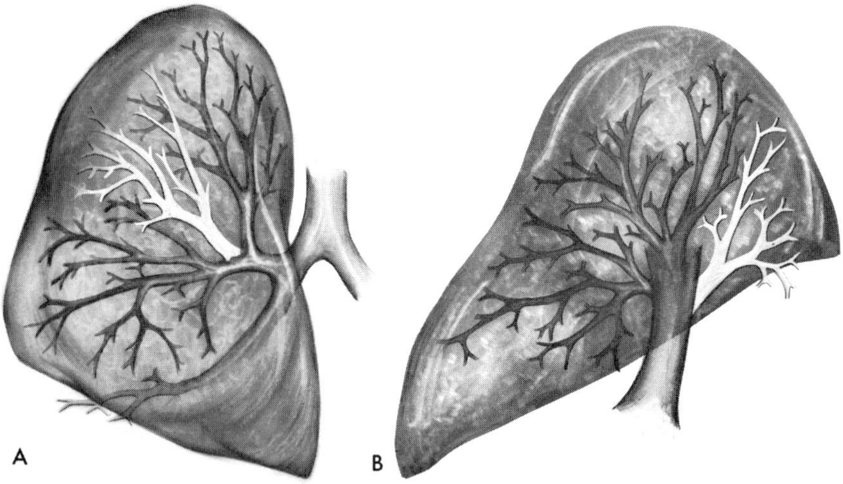

Figure 1–10. **Posterior Segmental Bronchus, Right Upper Lobe.** *A*, Frontal projection; *B*, lateral projection. This bronchus extends posteriorly, laterally, and somewhat superiorly to supply the posterolateral portion of the lobe.

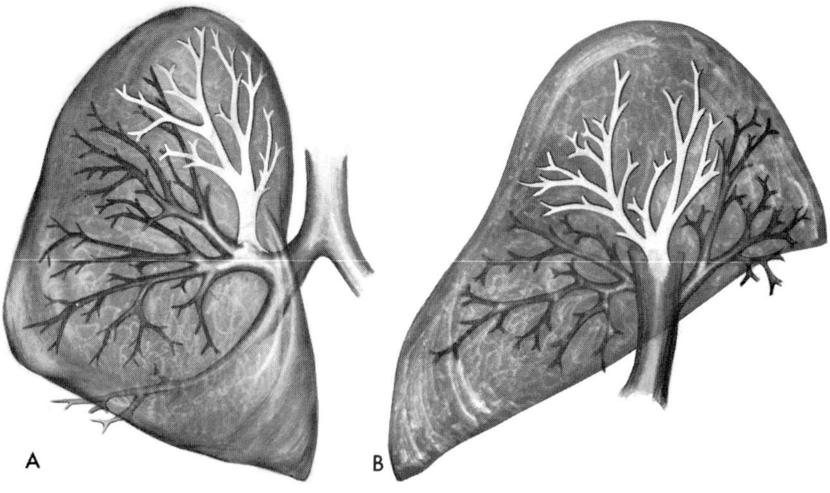

Figure 1–11. **Apical Segmental Bronchus, Right Upper Lobe.** *A*, Frontal projection; *B*, lateral projection. This bronchus supplies the superior paramediastinal zone, including the lung apex.

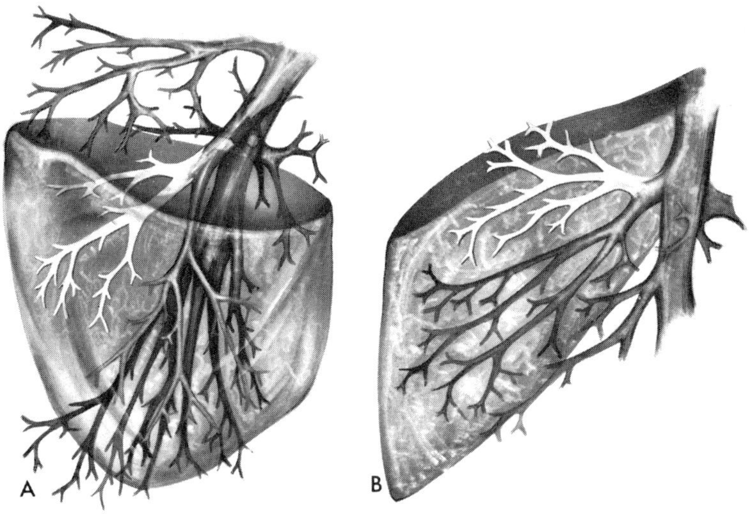

Figure 1–12. **Lateral Segmental Bronchus, Right Middle Lobe.** *A*, Frontal projection; *B*, lateral projection. This segment extends anterolaterally to supply that portion of the middle lobe which lies contiguous to the minor fissure and the anterior segment of the right upper lobe; its extreme lateral portion abuts against the chief fissure.

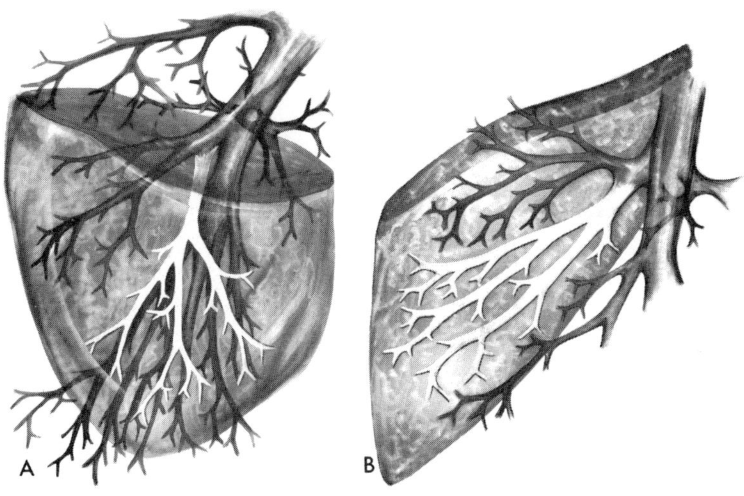

Figure 1–13. **Medial Segmental Bronchus, Right Middle Lobe.** *A*, Frontal projection; *B*, lateral projection. This bronchus extends anteromedially to supply the portion of the middle lobe which is contiguous to the heart and to the lower portion of the chief fissure.

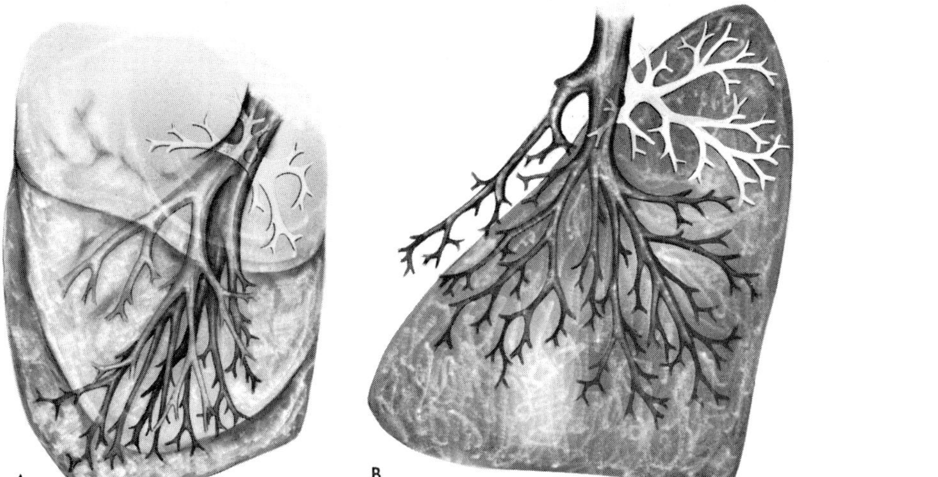

A B

Figure 1–14. **Superior Segmental Bronchus, Right Lower Lobe.** *A,* Frontal projection; *B,* lateral projection. Usually this bronchus has three subsegments which extend superiorly, laterally, and inferiorly to supply the apical region of the lower lobe.

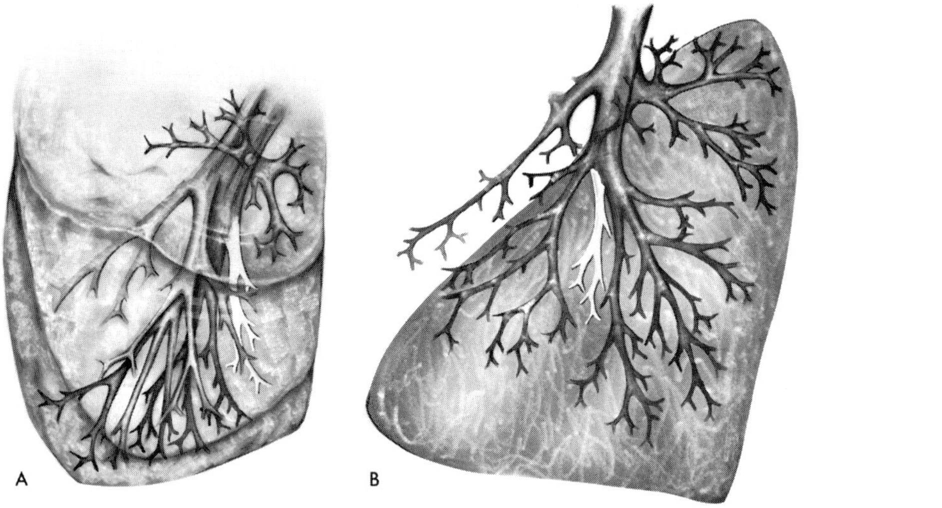

A B

Figure 1–15. **Medial Basal Bronchus, Right Lower Lobe.** *A,* Frontal projection; *B,* lateral projection. This is the first branch of the lower-lobe bronchus beyond the superior segmental bronchus; it is the smallest of the basal segments and the most medial in frontal projection. It arises from the medial aspect of the lower-lobe bronchus to supply the anteromedial portion of the lower lobe contiguous to the posterior portion of the heart and the lower end of the chief fissure.

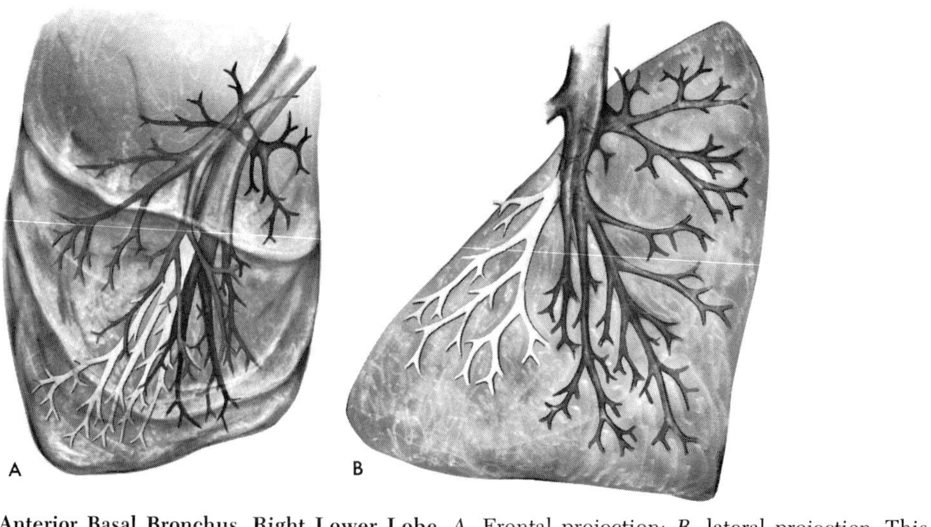

A B

Figure 1–16. **Anterior Basal Bronchus, Right Lower Lobe.** *A,* Frontal projection; *B,* lateral projection. This bronchus is the most lateral of the basal bronchi, extending anterolaterally into the costophrenic sulcus.

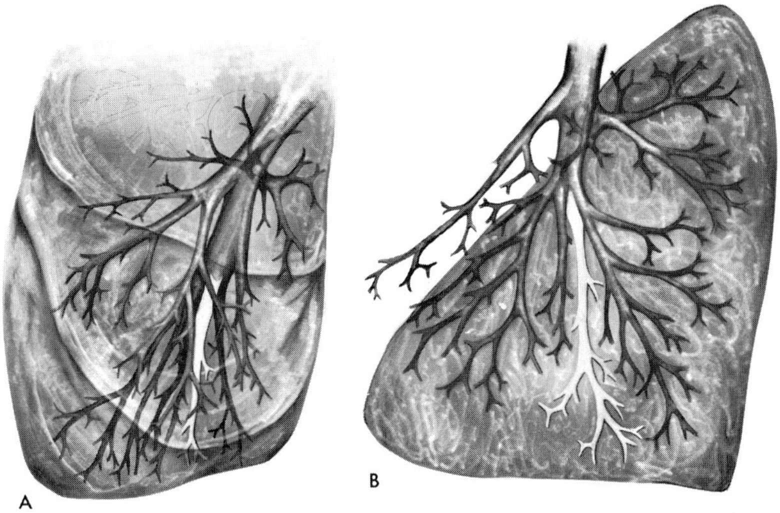

Figure 1–17. **Lateral Basal Bronchus, Right Lower Lobe.** *A*, Frontal projection; *B*, lateral projection. In frontal projection, this bronchus is projected just medial to the anterior basal bronchus; it extends laterally and slightly posteriorly to supply the portion of the lower lobe that lies behind the anterior basal bronchopulmonary segment. Neither the anterior nor the lateral bronchopulmonary segments relate to the major fissure, being separated from it by the medial segment.

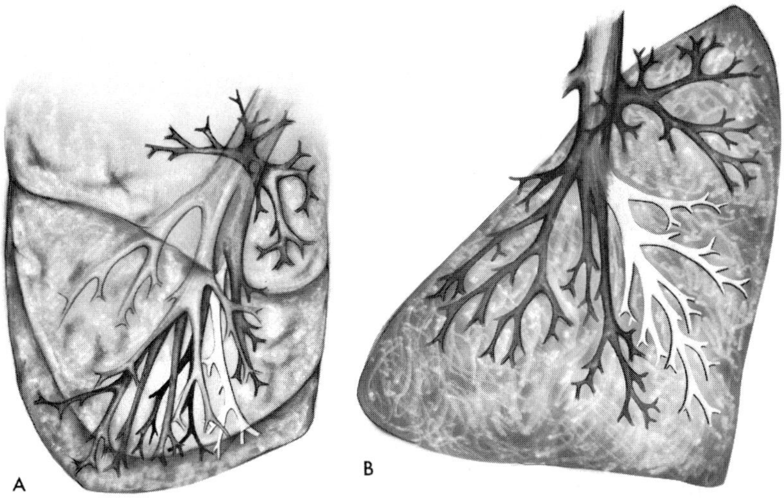

Figure 1–18. **Posterior Basal Bronchus, Right Lower Lobe.** *A*, Frontal projection; *B*, lateral projection. In frontal projection this bronchus appears between the lateral and medial basal bronchi; it supplies the posteroinferior portion of the lower lobe and extends into the posterior costophrenic gutter.

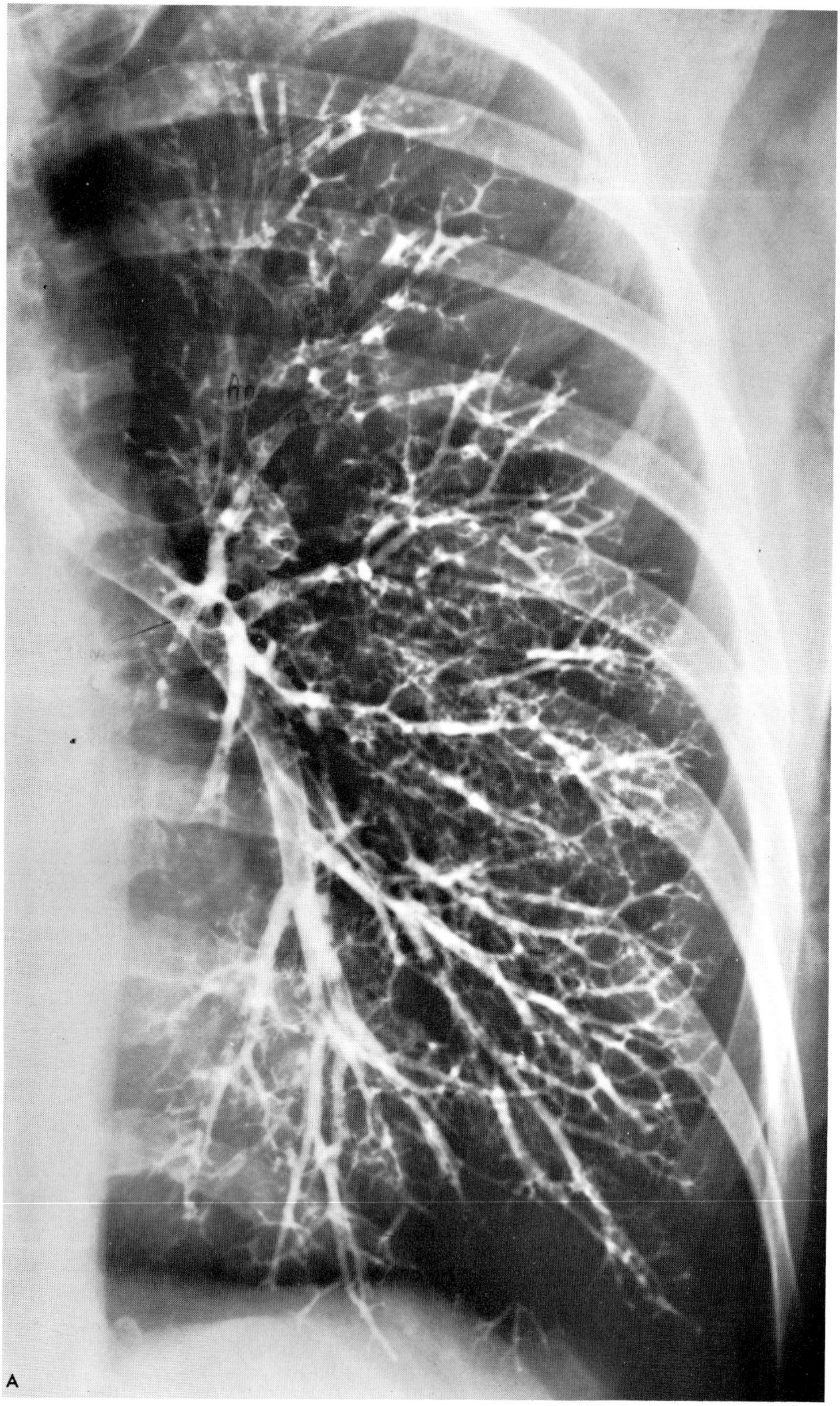

Figure 1–19. **Left Bronchial Tree (Frontal Projection).** *A*, Normal bronchogram of a 39-year-old woman.

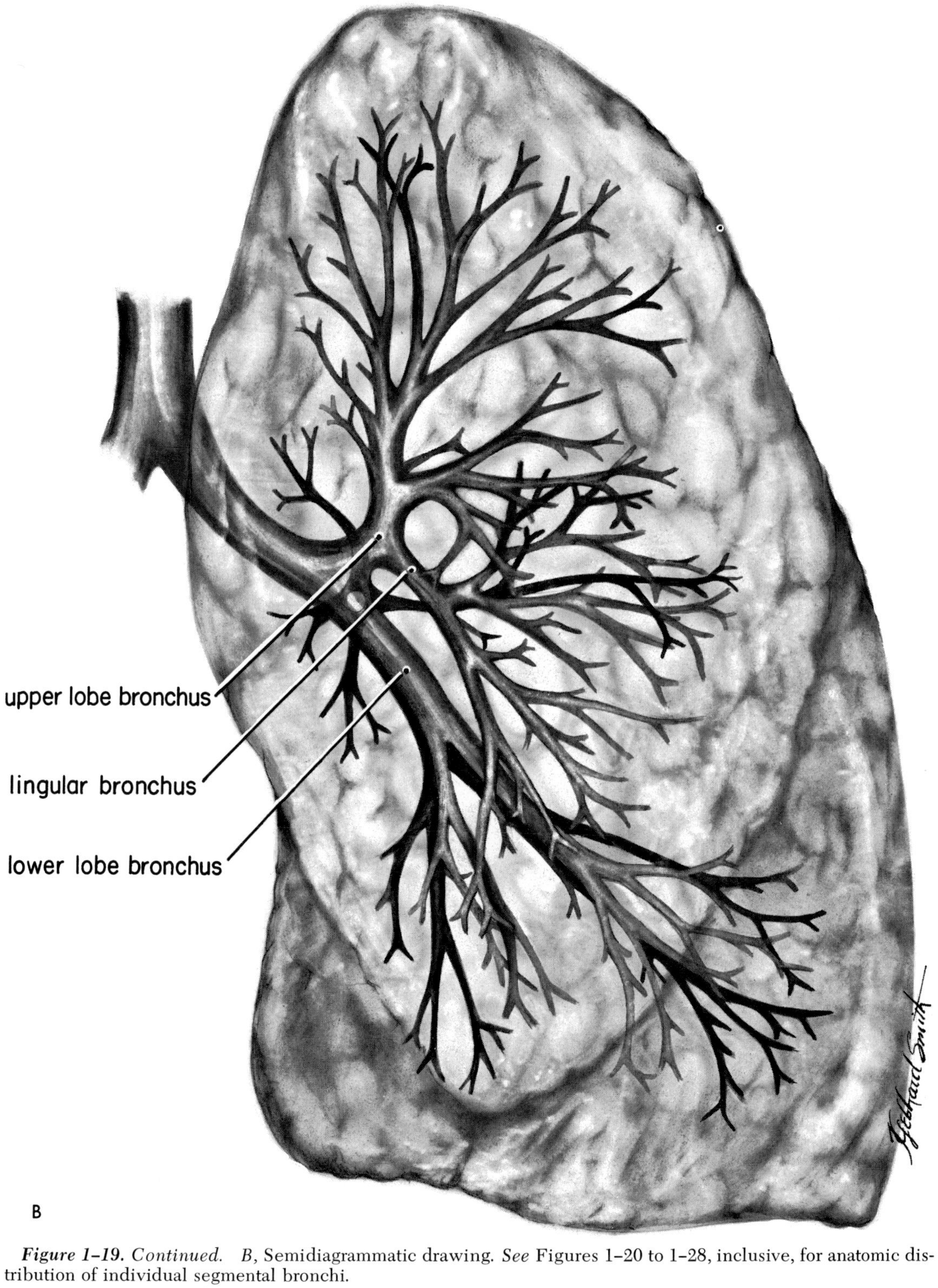

Figure 1–19. Continued. *B*, Semidiagrammatic drawing. *See* Figures 1–20 to 1–28, inclusive, for anatomic distribution of individual segmental bronchi.

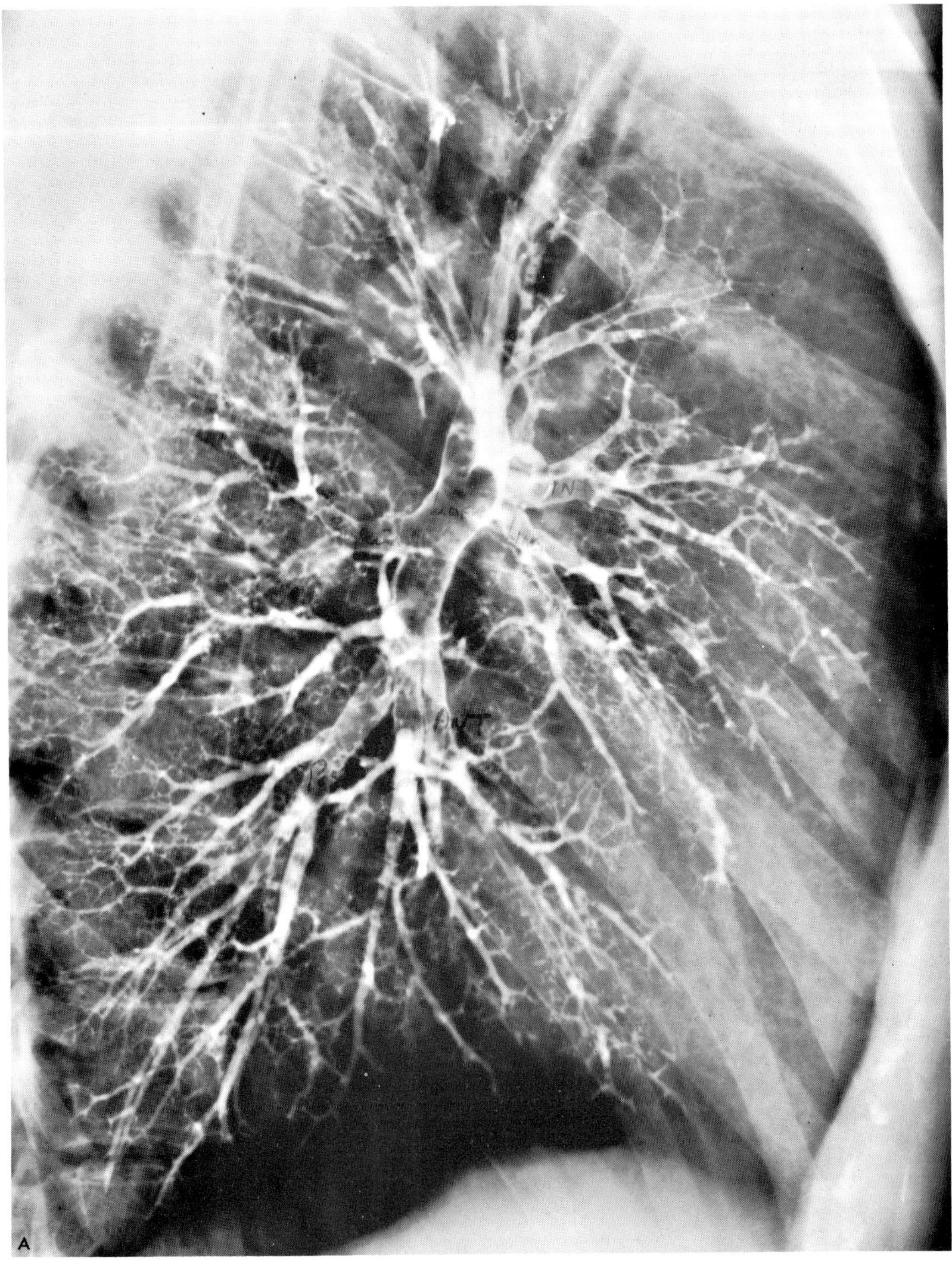

Figure 1–20. **Left Bronchial Tree (Lateral Projection).** *A,* Normal bronchogram of a 39-year-old woman.

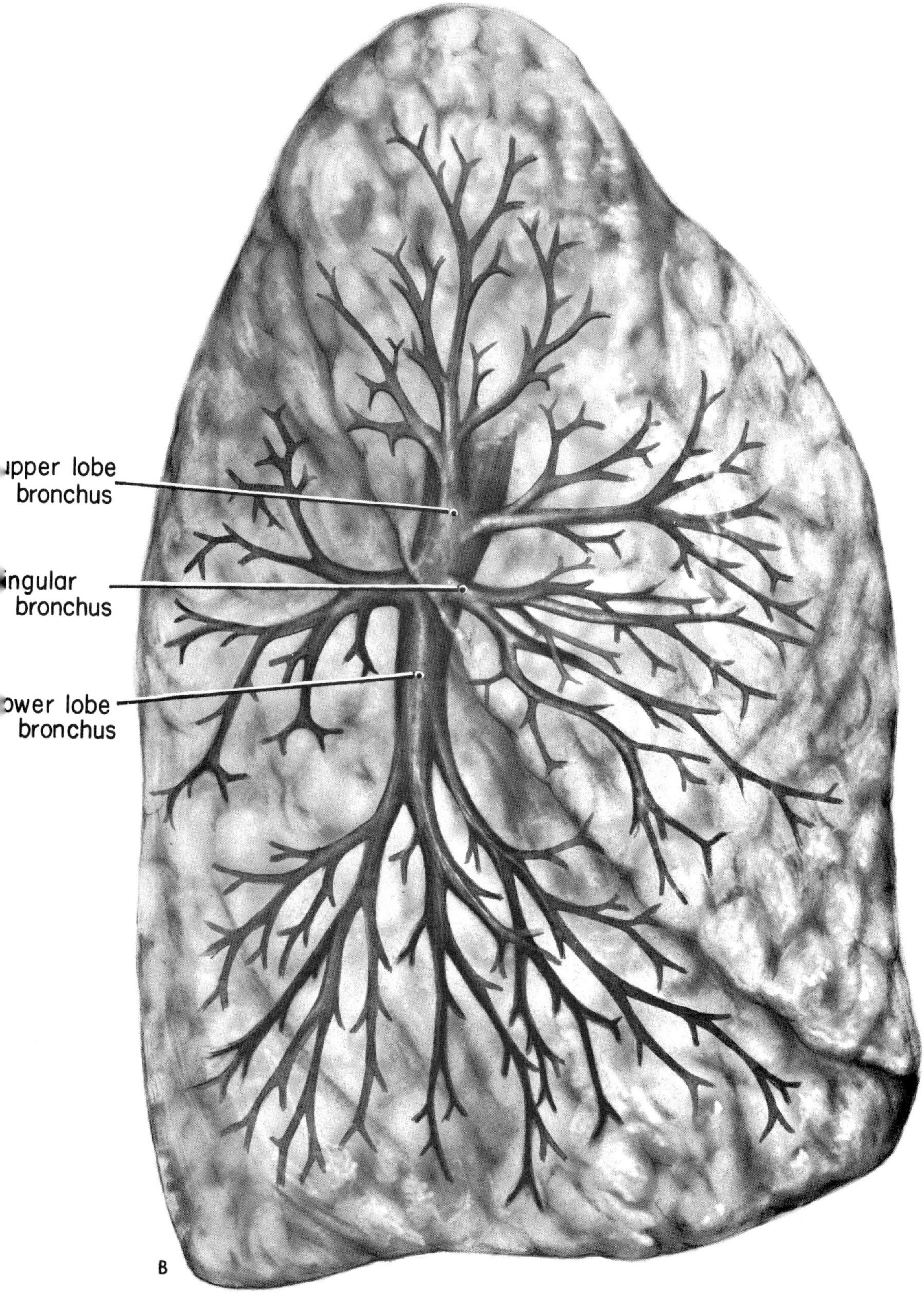

Figure 1–20. Continued. *B,* Semidiagrammatic drawing. *See* Figures 1–20 to 1–28, inclusive, for anatomic distribution of individual segmental bronchi.

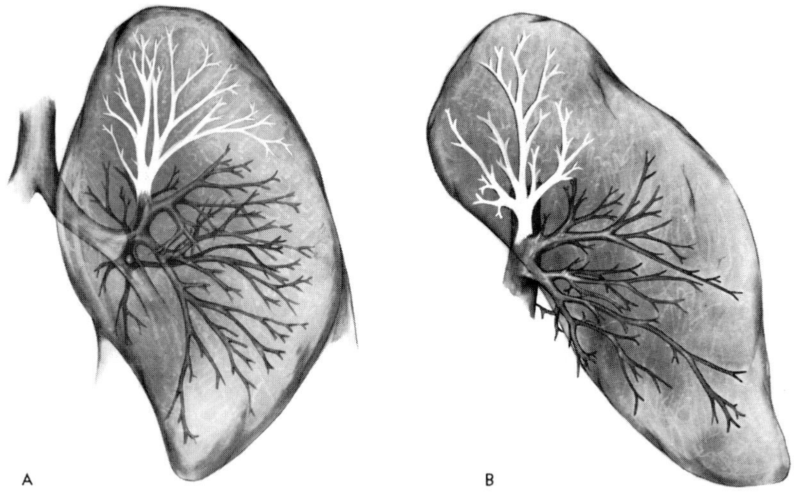

Figure 1–21. **Apical Posterior Bronchus, Left Upper Lobe.** *A,* Frontal projection; *B,* lateral projection. This bronchus bifurcates into apical and posterior segments which supply areas of the left upper lobe in a pattern similar to that of corresponding bronchi in the right upper lobe.

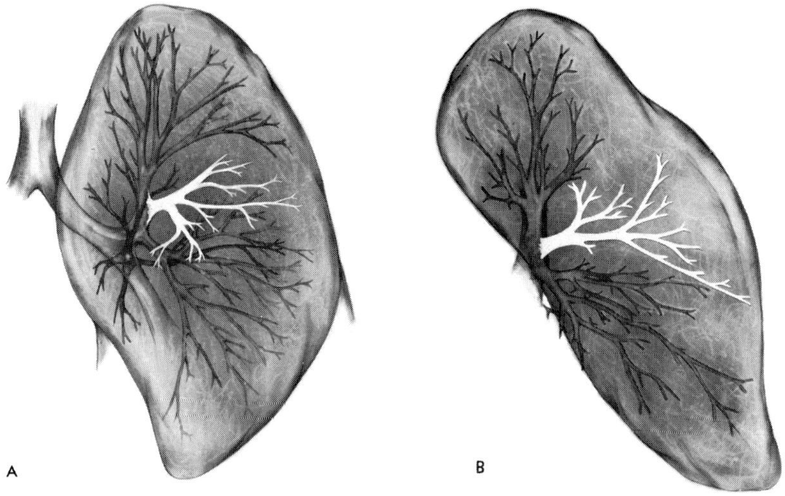

Figure 1–22. **Anterior Segmental Bronchus, Left Upper Lobe.** *A,* Frontal projection; *B,* lateral projection. The distribution is the same as in the right upper lobe.

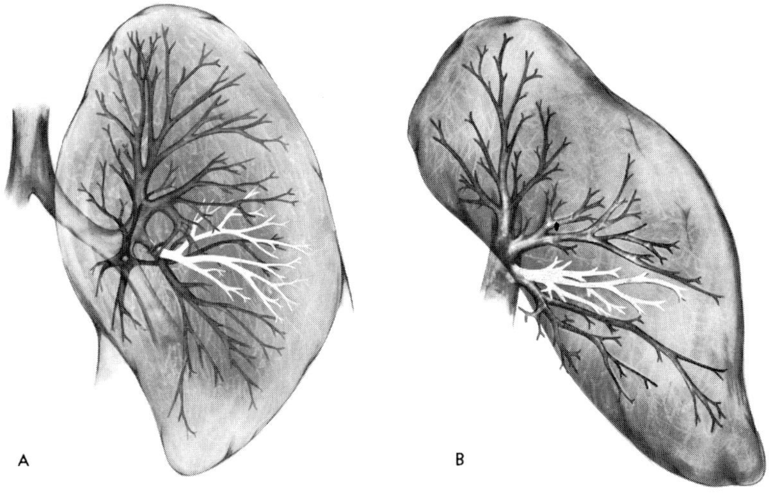

Figure 1–23. **Superior Segmental Bronchus, Lingula.** *A,* Frontal projection; *B,* lateral projection. This bronchus supplies the anterolateral portion of the lingula.

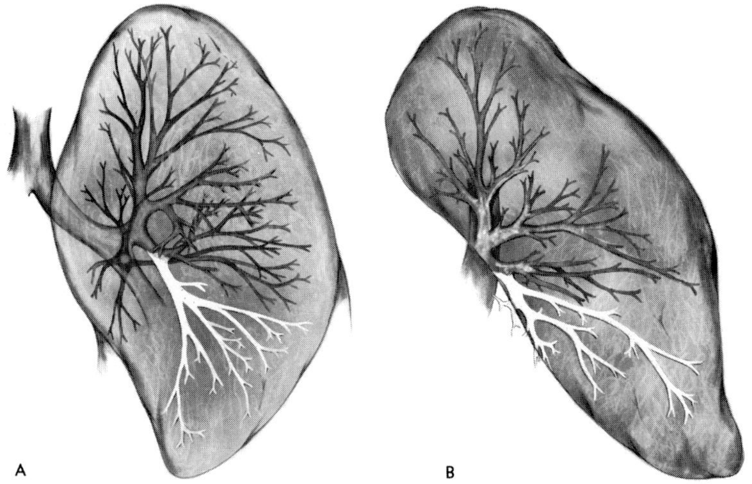

Figure 1–24. **Inferior Segmental Bronchus, Lingula.** *A,* Frontal projection; *B,* lateral projection. This segment supplies the inferomedial portion of the lingula contiguous to the left border of the heart. The lingula is somewhat larger in volume than the middle lobe of the right lung.

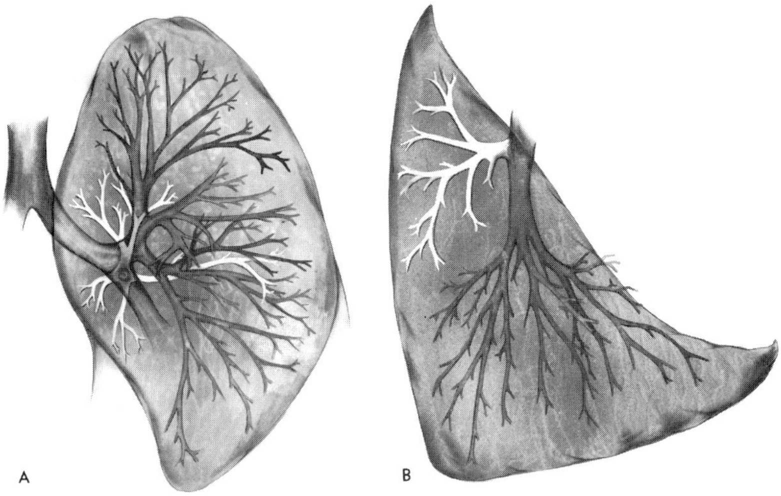

Figure 1–25. **Superior Segmental Bronchus, Left Lower Lobe.** *A,* Frontal projection; *B,* lateral projection. The distribution of this segment is similar to the corresponding segment of the right lower lobe.

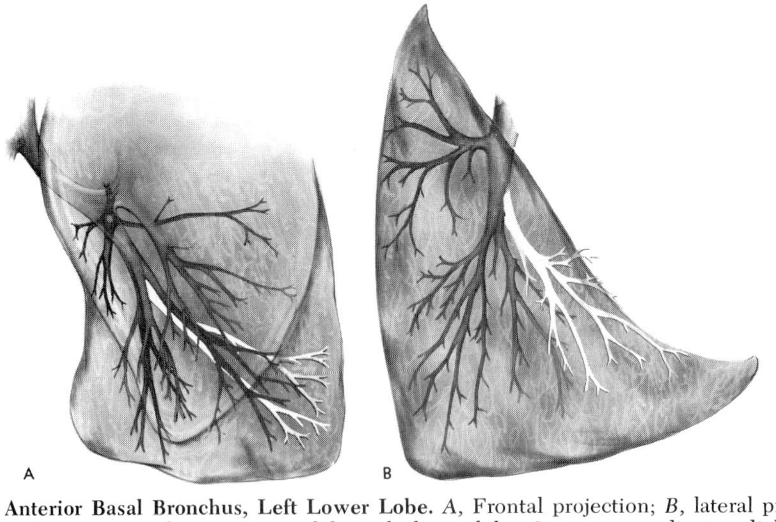

Figure 1–26. **Anterior Basal Bronchus, Left Lower Lobe.** *A,* Frontal projection; *B,* lateral projection. Distribution is similar to the corresponding segment of the right lower lobe. *See* text regarding medial basal bronchus.

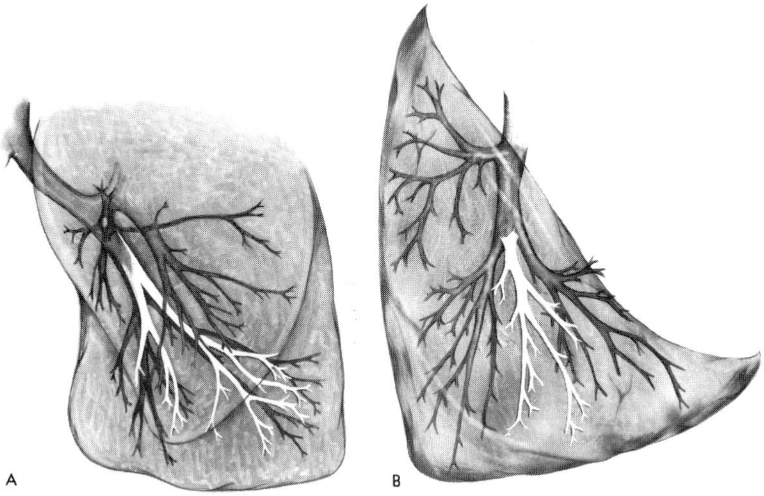

A B

Figure 1–27. **Lateral Basal Bronchus, Left Lower Lobe.** *A,* Frontal projection; *B,* lateral projection. Distribution is similar to the corresponding segment of the right lower lobe.

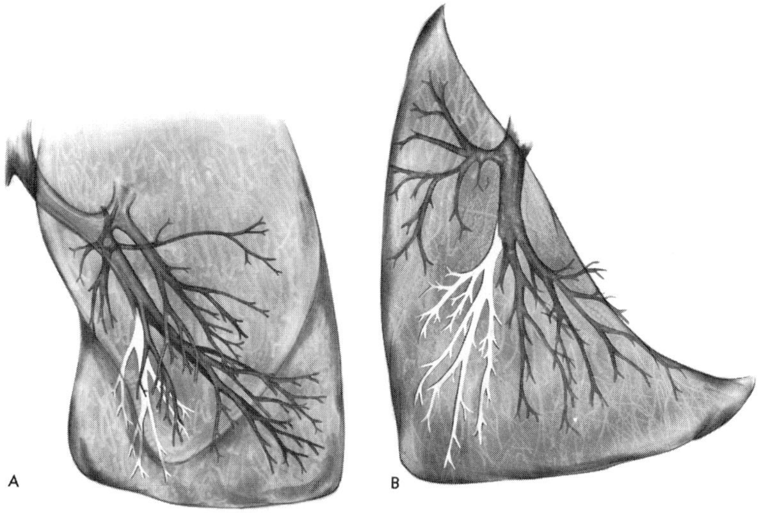

A B

Figure 1–28. **Posterior Basal Bronchus, Left Lower Lobe.** *A,* Frontal projection, *B,* lateral projection. Distribution is similar to the corresponding segment of the right lower lobe.

blood, nervous reflexes from the lungs themselves, chemoreceptors in blood vessels, and other reflexes from somatic and visceral tissues, including the cerebral cortex, act directly or indirectly on the respiratory center to produce movement of the diaphragm and intercostal muscles and, thus, an appropriate increase in ventilation. It follows that this increase in ventilation to satisfy the need for oxygen will be of no avail if there is not a parallel increase in circulating blood through the lungs to carry oxygen to the tissues. Accordingly, rate and stroke volume increase and, during exercise, for example, raise the cardiac output from, say, 5 liters/min to 25 to 30 liters/min.

Keeping in mind the chemical, nervous, and mechanical stimuli that act directly or indirectly on the respiratory center, cardiac muscle, airways, and pulmonary vessels and that vary the quantity of ventilation and perfusion of blood to the acinar unit, let us focus our attention on this unit, since it is here that the lung fulfills its role in the process of respiration. To do this we shall consider (1) alveolar gas and its composition, (2) the mechanism by which this gas is moved in and out of the acinus, (3) perfusion of the acinus, (4) the process of diffusion of gas in the acinar unit and across the alveolocapillary membrane to red blood cells, (5) the matching of blood flow with ventilation in the acinar unit, and the end result of these processes, (6) blood gases and H-ion concentration.

The Composition of Gas in Alveoli

The composition of this gas depends upon the rate and amount of oxygen removed and of carbon dioxide added by capillary blood (which, in turn, depends upon aerobic metabolism of tissues) and the quantity and quality of the gas which reaches the acinus through the tracheobronchial tree.

VENTILATION OF THE ACINUS. At sea level, air contains approximately 21 per cent oxygen and 79 per cent nitrogen and has an atmospheric pressure of 760 mm Hg; the amount of carbon dioxide and other gases is negligible and can be disregarded. The partial pressures of these gases are approximately 159 mm Hg for oxygen ($P_{O_2} = 21/100 \times 760$) and 601 mm Hg for nitrogen ($P_{N_2} = 79/100 \times 760$). As air is inhaled into the tracheobronchial tree, the body temperature fully saturates it with water vapor at a partial pressure of 47 mm Hg, so that the partial pressure of oxygen drops to 149 mm Hg ($(760 - 47) \times 21/100$). At sea level, therefore, the ventilation of alveoli depends upon the quantity of gas-containing oxygen, at a P_{O_2} of 149 mm Hg, that the thoracic "bellows" moves per minute into the acinus. Assuming that the conducting system is unobstructed, the quantity of gas reaching the alveoli depends upon the depth of respiration (tidal volume), the volume of the conducting system (dead-space gas which does not reach the alveoli), and the number of breaths per minute. If a subject moves 450 ml with each breath, has a respiratory dead space of 150 ml, and a respiratory rate of 15 per minute, his total minute ventilation is 6750 ml (450 ml $\times$ 15); since each breath contributes 300 ml of fresh air to the alveolar spaces, total alveolar ventilation is 300 $\times$ 15, or 4.5 liters/min. However, it must be realized that at the end of the previous expiration the dead space was filled not with atmospheric air but with expired air having a composition equivalent to that in the acinus. This means, therefore, that with each inspiration the first 150 ml reaching the alveoli has the composition of alveolar gas and the next 300 ml is inspired air saturated with water vapor; these two differently composed gas volumes probably mix instantly in the acini. The remaining 150 ml of the tidal volume of 450 ml is in the conducting system at the end of the inspiration (Figure 1–29).

ALVEOLAR-CAPILLARY GAS EXCHANGE. In addition to the contribution of ventilation to the composition of gas in the acinus, blood flow in the pulmonary capillaries varies the composition by the continuous removal of oxygen and addition of carbon dioxide. Obviously, as a result of these two dynamic processes, the composition of alveolar gas fluctuates, not only throughout the respiratory cycle but also from breath to breath and even from acinus to acinus (*see* page 50).

The quantity of oxygen removed from and carbon dioxide added to alveolar gas depends largely upon the metabolism of tissues. However, in man at rest—assuming that perfusion of blood and ventilation of acinar units are well matched—every 100 ml of blood allows approximately 5.6 ml of carbon dioxide to diffuse into the alveolar

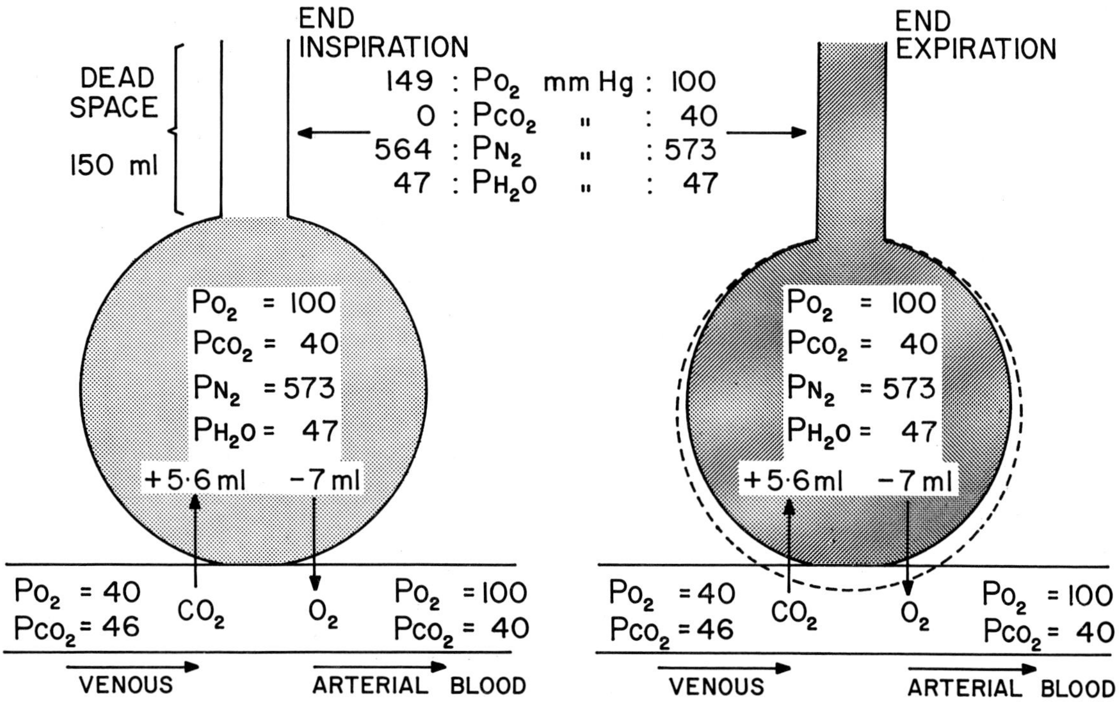

Figure 1–29. **A Diagram Portraying the Conducting System Leading to an Acinar Unit.** At the end of an inspiration of 450 ml of air, 150 ml of fresh air (saturated with water vapor) are situated within the conducting system and the remaining 300 ml have entered and mixed with alveolar gas. At end-expiration the conducting system (dead space) is filled with alveolar air. Carbon dioxide moves from the capillary blood to the alveolus and oxygen from the alveolus to the capillary blood so that the gas composition of alveolar gas and blood are altered. *See* text.

spaces. At the same time, 7 ml of oxygen leaves the acinar units and is carried away by each 100 ml of blood going to the tissues. The partial pressure of carbon dioxide (P_{CO_2}) in the acinus then is 40 mm Hg (713 × 5.6/100). The removal of oxygen, decreasing it from approximately 21 per cent to 14 per cent, gives a partial pressure of oxygen (P_{O_2}) of 100 mm Hg (713 × 14/100) (Figure 1–29).

SUMMARY. The composition of acinar gas varies with the metabolism of the tissues and the total alveolar ventilation. Increasing activity of tissues results in greater oxygen consumption and carbon dioxide production, which in turn lower the P_{O_2} and raise the P_{CO_2} of the mixed venous blood returning to the lungs. The total alveolar ventilation depends upon tidal volume and respiratory rate.

Mechanics of Acinar Ventilation

Movement of atmospheric air down the conducting system to the acinar unit requires a certain force or pressure to overcome the "elastic" recoil of the lungs and the thoracic cage, the frictional resistance of pulmonary tissue and chest wall, and the resistance of the airways themselves. This pressure is produced by contraction of the muscles of inspiration, mainly the diaphragm, to a lesser extent the external intercostal muscles, and, in circumstance requiring greatly increased ventilation, the accessory respiratory muscles in the neck. At the end of inspiratory effort the inspiratory muscles relax; expiration usually occurs passively as the "elastic" parenchyma recoils to its resting state. If elastic recoil is defective, or if the conducting system is obstructed, expiratory muscles, particularly the abdominal mucles, come into play. This occurs also when large quantities of air are moved rapidly in and out of the chest.

Thus, air is brought to the acinus by the contraction of respiratory muscles, which exert a force or pressure to overcome the elastic recoil and frictional resistance of lung and thoracic cage, as well as the airway resistance of the tracheobronchial tree.

"ELASTIC" RECOIL OF LUNG PARENCHYMA AND THE THORACIC CAGE. The pressure in the pleural space normally is subatmospheric, *i.e.*, 4 to 5 cm H_2O below that of the atmosphere. If air is introduced into this "space" and the visceral and parietal layers of pleura are allowed to separate, the lungs and the thoracic cage assume new positions, the former collapsing and the latter enlarging (Figure 1–30). This is the "elastic" recoil which is overcome by contraction of the respiratory muscles and expansion of the thoracic cage and which represents the main mechanical impedance during quiet breathing.

On inspiration, the respiratory muscles act *initially* to overcome the "elastic" recoil of the lungs only; the thoracic cage, with an elastic recoil which allows a more expanded state, actually aids pulmonary inflation. As inspiration continues, the chest wall goes beyond its resting position and the force of muscular contraction then is exerted against the recoil of both lung and thoracic cage. As the cage expands, the intrapleural pressure becomes more subatmospheric, the acini and conducting tubes enlarge, gaseous pressure in the alveoli decreases in relation to atmospheric pressure at the mouth, and air moves down the conducting system. The force or pressure exerted on the lungs by muscle contraction overcomes both elastic recoil and flow resistance; this pressure is measurable since it is reflected in the degree of change in intrapleural pressure. Measurement is made directly or, more conveniently, by use of an intraesophageal balloon which reflects changes in intrapleural pressure. The relationship of the change in intrapleural pressure to the volume of gas which moves into the lungs is expressed as liters/cm H_2O and is known as lung compliance. To distinguish the force or pressure needed to overcome "elastic" recoil from that required to overcome resistance in the air-

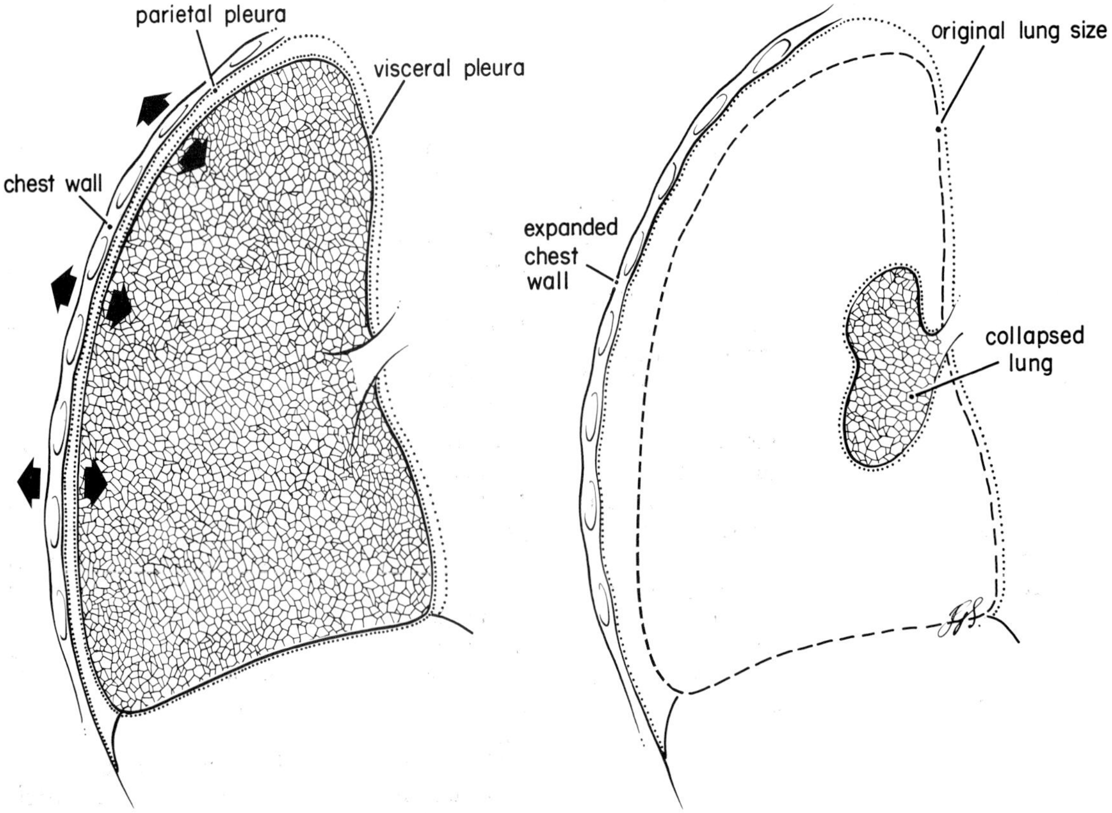

Figure 1–30. **Elastic Recoil of Lung and Cage.** Arrows indicate the elastic recoil of lung and thoracic cage. Introduction of air into the pleural cavity causes lung and thoracic cage to assume "resting" positions.

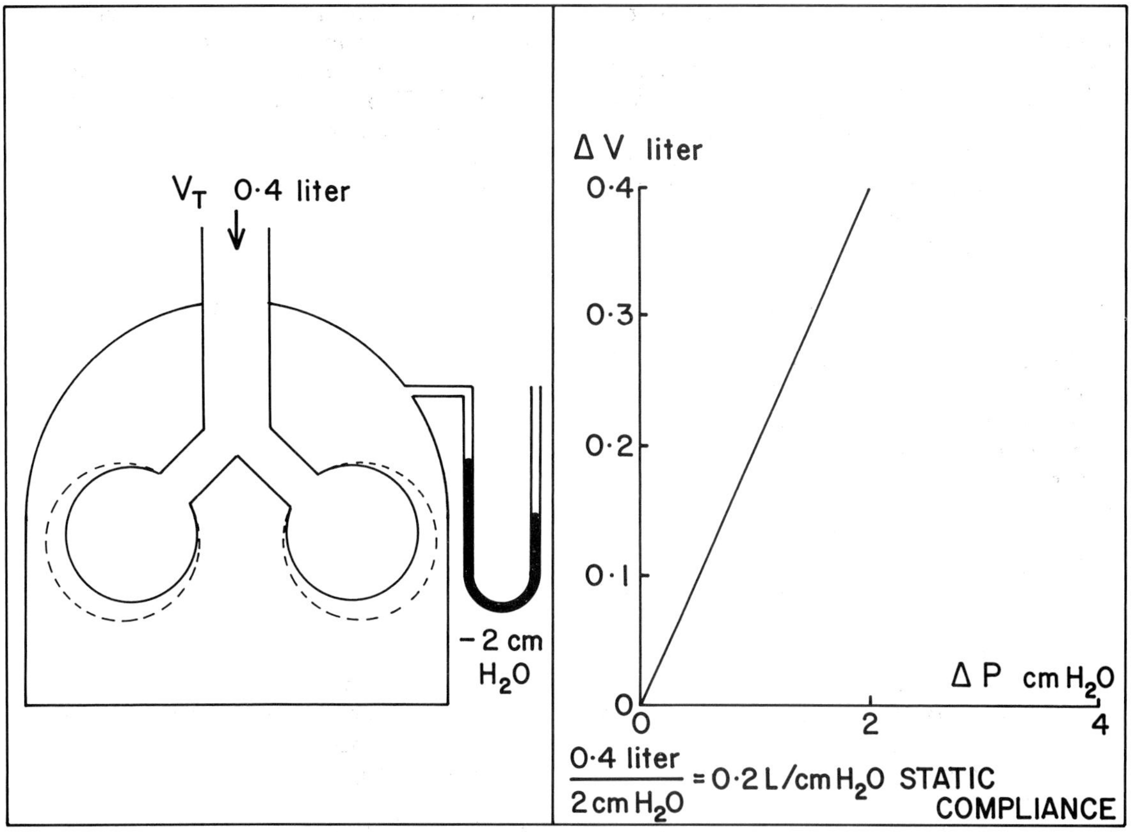

Figure 1–31. **Pressure–Volume Relationships.** A change of 2 cm H_2O in pleural pressure (ΔP) results in a volume change (ΔV) of 0.4 L of tidal air (V_T) in two hypothetical acini. The diagram on the right depicts the change in volume of 0.4 L and the change in pressure of 2 cm H_2O. The static compliance in this example is 0.2 L/cm H_2O.

ways and lung tissue, measurement is made with breathing suspended, when flow in the bronchi ceases and flow resistance is eliminated. Under these conditions, only the pressure required to overcome elasticity is measured. The resulting volume change affected by the pressure change is the static compliance (Figure 1–31). As the normal lung becomes more inflated it becomes less compliant; for this reason it is more informative to express compliance as the change in intrapleural pressure required to produce a volume change at a specific degree of lung inflation, generally functional residual capacity (FRC). Edema and fibrotic or granulomatous infiltration render the lungs stiffer and less compliant, so that more pressure is required to move a given volume of gas; or, to put it differently, a given pressure moves a smaller volume. When the elastic architecture of the lung is faulty, as in emphysema, a given pressure may actually produce a greater volume change than in the normal lung, and in such a case compliance is increased.

"Elastic" recoil of the lung has been attributed in part to the peculiar arrangement of collagenous and elastic fibers.[42, 43] The helical structure of this fibrous network gives the lungs an elastic behavior similar to that of a coil spring. However, tissue elasticity is not the only component of the elastic recoil of the lungs. This was first indicated by the work of von Neergaard[44] in 1929, who measured the pressure-volume relationships of a fluid-distended lung and an air-distended lung and found less elastic recoil in the former: less pressure change was required to fully distend the fluid-filled lung than the air-filled lung. Von Neergaard deduced that a surface tension, a force which tended to contract alveolar spaces and to resist expansion, existed in each alveolus between its lining and its gas content. He suggested that this surface tension accounted for most of the lung's elastic recoil and that it was eliminated when gas was replaced by liquid.

SURFACE TENSION AND SURFACTANT. Subsequent work indicates that the surface tension at the air-liquid interface of the alveolar wall is variable, depending upon whether the lungs are inflating or deflating. The layer lining the alveoli contains a substance which can lower surface tension as alveolar spaces decrease in size during expiration.[45-49] Perhaps surface tension is best exemplified by a child's bubble pipe: the bubble on the mouth of the bowl tends to retract into the pipe and a distending force is necessary to counteract this effect.[50] A soap bubble, however, has a constant surface tension. An analogous but somewhat different situation exists in relation to the acinus on the end of the terminal bronchiole or the alveoli on the end of the alveolar duct. As distending pressure decreases and the alveoli become smaller in expiration, the collapse that occurred in the child's bubble pipe is prevented by the presence in the lining membrane of a surface-active substance, or surfactant, which can lower surface tension almost to zero.

It is believed that deep breaths are required from time to time to replenish the surface-active substance and that continued shallow breathing may eventually lead to collapse.[51] The implications of the effect of surface tension and surfactant on the capillary circulation are considerable; they are discussed in a subsequent section (*see* page 46). Surfactant is generally considered to be secreted by alveolar corner cells. A recent report indicates that surfactant originates in Clara cells in the distal bronchioles, and that subsequently it is taken up from the alveoli by alveolar corner cells.[184] It probably is a lipoprotein whose chief lipid is alpha dipalmitoyl-lecithin, a substance which may be in osmophilic lamellar inclusions in certain alveolar epithelial cells.[52]

Under experimental conditions it has been shown that occlusion of blood supply to a lung, occlusion of a main bronchus, or the prolonged inhalation of high concentrations of oxygen or carbon dioxide results in a loss of surfactant and the development of atelectasis. In addition, there are at least three clinical conditions in which loss of surfactant appears to be responsible for lung collapse: (1) hyaline membrane disease of the newborn;[53] (2) atelectasis in patients who have died after use of an artificial heart-lung system during open-heart surgery;[54] and (3) after hyperbaric oxygen therapy.[200] Experimental evidence indicates that this substance becomes inactivated whenever circulation to the acinus is inadequate or when plasma proteins escape into the alveoli. Several reviews of this subject have been published.[50, 55-57]

RESISTANCE OF THE AIRWAYS. During quiet breathing, most of the work of the respiratory muscles is required to overcome elastic recoil; when ventilation becomes more rapid, flow increases and increased work is necessary to overcome resistance in the conducting airways. Resistance increases in direct proportion to the length of a tubular conducting system, so that twice as much pressure is required to maintain the same flow in a tube doubled in length. However, reduction in the radius of a tube by one-half requires a 16-fold increase in pressure to maintain the same flow. These principles of laminar flow pertain to rigid, smooth tubes. Bronchial flow and airway resistance are more complicated: not only are the bronchial tubes irregular but they branch frequently and vary in caliber throughout the respiratory cycle. These additional features create turbulence which adds to resistance. Resistance is different during inspiration and expiration and varies with both lung volume and flow rate. Because of the nature of the branching of the bronchial tree, the total cross-sectional area becomes markedly increased with each new generation beyond the segmental bronchi, with the result that resistance is much less in the bronchioles than in the bronchi (*see* Table 1–1, page 9).

Anatomic differences between the larger cartilaginous bronchi and the smaller membranous bronchioles suggest a difference in function of these two portions of the conducting system which is supported by certain physiologic studies.[58, 59] Bronchi which contain cartilage remain patent after removal from the body; bronchioles, however, because of their content of elastic and muscle tissue, collapse in similar circumstances.[60] During life these cartilages not only maintain patency of the larger airways during expiration but also prevent overdistention during maximal inspiration.[58] These two portions of the conducting system differ not only in the construction of their walls but also in the fact that they occupy different thoracic-cage "compartments," which are separated by a strong elastic limiting membrane.[15] The cartilage-containing airways appear to have a potential space around them[22] and are affected more by changes in transpulmonary pressure (the difference between pressure at the mouth and intrapleural pressure) than by changes in the lung volume.[38, 59, 61] The bronchioles, on the other hand, lie on the other side of a limiting membrane which fuses with the bronchial walls at the point where the cartilage disappears.[15] They lie within the lobule, tightly connected to the pulmonary parenchyma, and the patency of their lumina is influenced by changes in lung volume.

During expiration, as lung volume becomes smaller and intrapleural pressure becomes less subatmospheric, resistance in both bronchi and bronchioles increases. Most of the increase in resistance, however, is in the bronchi and is due to their bronchomotor tone. In the absence of bronchomotor tone, there is very little increase in resistance as lung volume decreases until the lung volume becomes very small.[62]

In addition to these passive forces acting on the conducting system and causing increase or decrease in resistance, there are active stimuli to both bronchodilatation and bronchoconstriction. These are mediated through nervous pathways or by the action of chemicals, either on the receptor sites for postganglionic fibers or through direct action on smooth muscle. The action of histamine is of particular interest: injection of this substance into the pulmonary artery causes constriction of alveolar-duct sphincters and, thus, expulsion of air from acinar units. It is thought that microemboli act by the release of histamine, which causes closure of the alveolar ducts. This selective response to histamine when injected into the pulmonary artery reflects the fact that the blood supply to the acinus is from pulmonary arterioles, whereas the remainder of the airways is supplied by bronchial arterioles.[63]

Reflex local bronchoconstriction occurs when adjacent major pulmonary arteries are obstructed, constituting what appears to be a compensatory mechanism to divert ventilation to perfused areas.[64, 65] The operation of this mechanism may be prevented by the inhalation of 3 to 5 per cent carbon dioxide and it is thought that bronchoconstriction occurring in these circumstances is due to the reduced P_{CO_2}.[153]

A sudden increase in resistance, as during attacks of asthma, prolongs expiration and thereby prevents complete emptying of the acinar unit; the next inspiration enlarges the unit and thus increases the functional residual capacity. This increase in lung volume augments elastic recoil to supply greater expiratory force.

Obstruction in the airways is not always the result of constriction of smooth muscle, and may be due to mucus in the bronchi or bronchioles or, as in emphysema, to "weak" walls. In this condition airway resistance is increased both because of loss of elastic tissue to hold open the smaller bronchi or bronchioles and because of the development of a high intrapleural pressure in an attempt to force air out of the alveolar spaces.

Tissue Resistance. During movement of the chest, in addition to airway resistance, tissue resistance is present; this is caused by displacement of lung tissue itself, the rib cage, the diaphragm, and the abdominal contents. It is generally thought that in a healthy person, tissue resistance accounts for about 20 per cent and airway resistance 80 per cent of total pulmonary resistance. This, however, may be an overestimate.[201] Tissue resistance is increased when the lung is infiltrated by granulomatous, fibrotic, or malignant tissue. During expiration some of the elastic force is used to overcome this additional frictional resistance, and, since there is less force available to overcome resistance in the conducting system, expiration is slowed.

Summary. The force required to overcome the "elastic recoil" and the resistance of lungs, bronchial tubes, and thoracic cage is measured as a pressure in centimeters of water. The relationship of pressure to volume of gas moved in and out of the lungs is known as compliance and is expressed as liters/cm H_2O. Compliance is decreased when the lung is made stiffer by fibrotic or granulomatous infiltration; it is increased when pulmonary elastic recoil is reduced, as in emphysema. Elastic recoil is only partially due to the elasticity of lung parenchyma. A major component is dependent upon alveolar surface tension, which increases with inspiration and decreases with expiration; this tension is modified by a substance known as surfactant, which is present in the alveoli.

During quiet breathing most of the work of the respiratory muscles is required to overcome elastic recoil. During rapid respirations the increase in flow, the irregularity of the bronchi (which produces turbulence), and the bronchomotor tone add a significant impedance to ventilation. Bronchospasm or mucus in the airways add to this resistance. Loss of elastic support to the smaller bronchi and bronchioles and development of a high intrapleural pressure during expiration are responsible for the severe degree of airway resistance which develops in emphysema. Parenchymal and thoracic-wall tissues also create a resistance to respiration and this may be considerable when diseased lungs are diffusely infiltrated.

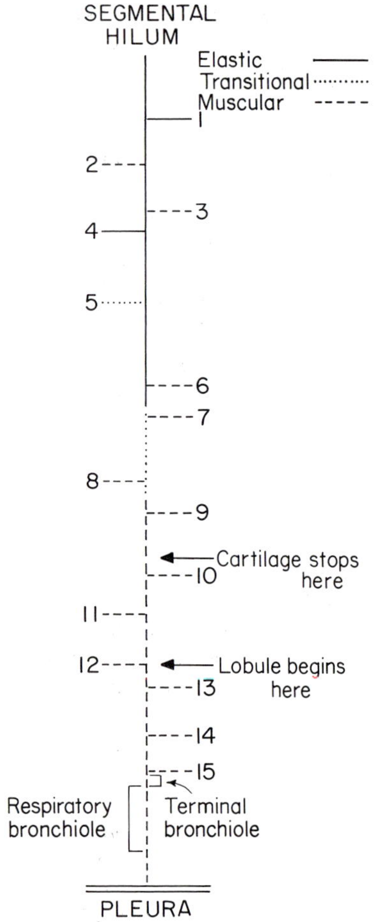

Figure 1–32. **Structure of the Pulmonary Arteries.** Diagrammatic representation (drawn to scale) of the full length of an anterior basal segmental artery. The structure of the artery is related to bronchial generations, and only conventional branches are included—those which accompany airways. (Reproduced with the permission of the Editor of *Clinical Radiology* and of the authors—Elliott, F. M., and Reid, Lynne: Some new facts about the pulmonary artery and its branching pattern. Clin. Radiol., *16*:193-198, 1965.)

THE PULMONARY VASCULAR SYSTEM

MORPHOLOGY

The pulmonary arterial system accompanies the bronchial tree and divides with it, a branch always accompanying the appropriate bronchial division; these have been termed "conventional" branches. However, it was shown recently that many accessory branches of the pulmonary artery arise at points other than corresponding bronchial divisions.[66] These accessory branches outnumber the conventional ones; they originate throughout the length of the arterial tree and are most frequent peripherally.

The pulmonary arterial system may be conveniently divided into three types—elastic, transitional, and muscular. The arteries that accompany bronchi are elastic, and those that run with nonrespiratory bronchioles are muscular: the former vessels have a well-defined internal and external elastic lamina, with seven or more elastic laminae between, and the latter have an internal and an external elastic lamina with less than four elastic laminae between. Vessels that have intermediate amounts of elastic tissue are termed "transitional" arteries. The number of generations of the types of artery differs in various pathways. In the anterior basal segmental artery (Figure 1–32), elastic arteries stop at about the sixth order, followed by two orders of transitional arteries coinciding with the end of the cartilage in the bronchi. Beyond this the vessels are muscular in type. Many muscular vessels arise proximally from elastic vessels which correspond to side branches along lateral pathways of the bronchial tree. The muscular arteries measure about 2000μ in diameter at their point of origin and diminish to about 100μ at the level of the terminal bronchiole. The walls become progressively thinner, with loss of elastic lamina and muscle. Beyond the level of the terminal bronchioles the arteries lose their continuous muscle coat and become arterioles, with a single elastic lamina. Within the acinus, arterioles continue to divide and accompany their respective branches of the respiratory tree to the level of the alveolar sacs. Many accessory branches are given off to supply the walls of the acinar pathways and the alveoli. These branches, as well as those which terminate around the alveolar sacs, are sometimes called precapillary arterioles; they break up to form the capillary network of the alveoli themselves. The capillary network of the alveoli is the densest in the body, and the area of capillary surface is only slightly less than that of the alveolar surface.

The *bronchial arteries*, usually three in number (sometimes more), are inconstant in origin; they may arise from the aorta or from any of the first three intercostal, subclavian, or internal mammary arteries. They supply the bronchial wall as far as the terminal bronchioles, forming one arterial plexus in the peribronchium and another in the tunica propria. The bronchial arteries also supply the tracheobronchial lymph nodes, the midesophagus, and the mediastinal pleura. Distal branches anastomose with one another and with the systemic arterial supply of the pericardium. In some forms of bronchiectasis the bronchial artery system is greatly hypertrophied and may carry significant quantities of blood.

The *pulmonary venous radicles* arise from capillaries distal to the alveolar meshwork and from the capillary network of the pleura. Histologically, venules are indistinguishable from arterioles other than by their position. The venous system drains via the interlobular septa, and thus does not accompany the corresponding bronchial or arterial tree. A bronchial vein plexus, which corresponds to the bronchial artery plexus, extends proximally from the level of the respiratory bronchioles and connects at intervals with the pulmonary veins; most of the veins of the intrapulmonary bronchi drain into the pulmonary veins. The venous drainage of the large bronchi and the tracheal bifurcation form a few small trunks (bronchial veins) that drain into the azygos system and receive branches from the mediastinum. Connections exist between these veins and the intrabronchial venous plexus.

Arteriovenous Anastomoses

Precapillary anastomoses between pulmonary arteries and veins, and between bronchial and pulmonary arteries, may be found in disease; it is not certain whether they occur in the normal lung. Data concerning pulmonary arteriovenous anastomoses are conflicting; some authors claim to have found connections up to 420μ in diameter, whereas others have seen none. Liebow[67] recently reviewed this controversial subject. Turner-Warwick[68] found no anastomoses between systemic and pulmonary arteries in normal lung, but in diseased lungs she observed subpleural and intrapleural anastomoses that appeared to represent enlargement of pre-existing channels.

Roentgenology

The *main pulmonary artery* curves upward from the pulmonic valve to form a segment of the left border of the heart. At the level of the carina and slightly to the left of the midline it bifurcates into right and left branches (Figure 1–33). The right branch is almost horizontal in position, and divides into two main branches while still within the mediastinum and before reaching the hilum; the left curves sharply *upward* and backward as it passes into the left hilum, which, therefore, is situated slightly higher and more posterior than the right. In a series of 500 normal subjects in whom the relative levels of the hila were assessed, the left hilum was higher than the right in 97 per cent, the majority (80.4 per cent) showing a difference in level of 0.75 to 2.25 cm.[69] In 3 per cent the hila were at the same level and in none was the right higher than the left. The right hilum usually is projected in the plane of the sixth interspace posteriorly.

The *right pulmonary artery* lies posterior to the aorta and the superior vena cava and anterior to the right main bronchus (Figures 1–33 and 1–34). Its superior branch, the truncus anterior, supplies most of the upper lobe. It curves superiorly and anteriorly over the upper-lobe bronchus and then divides into three branches which follow the anterior, apical, and posterior segmental bronchi. Jefferson[70] found that in 90 per cent of patients a portion of the posterior bronchopulmonary segment is supplied by a separate arterial branch which arises from the descending artery distal to the take-off of the truncus anterior.

The inferior of the two pulmonary arteries in the right hilum (the interlobar

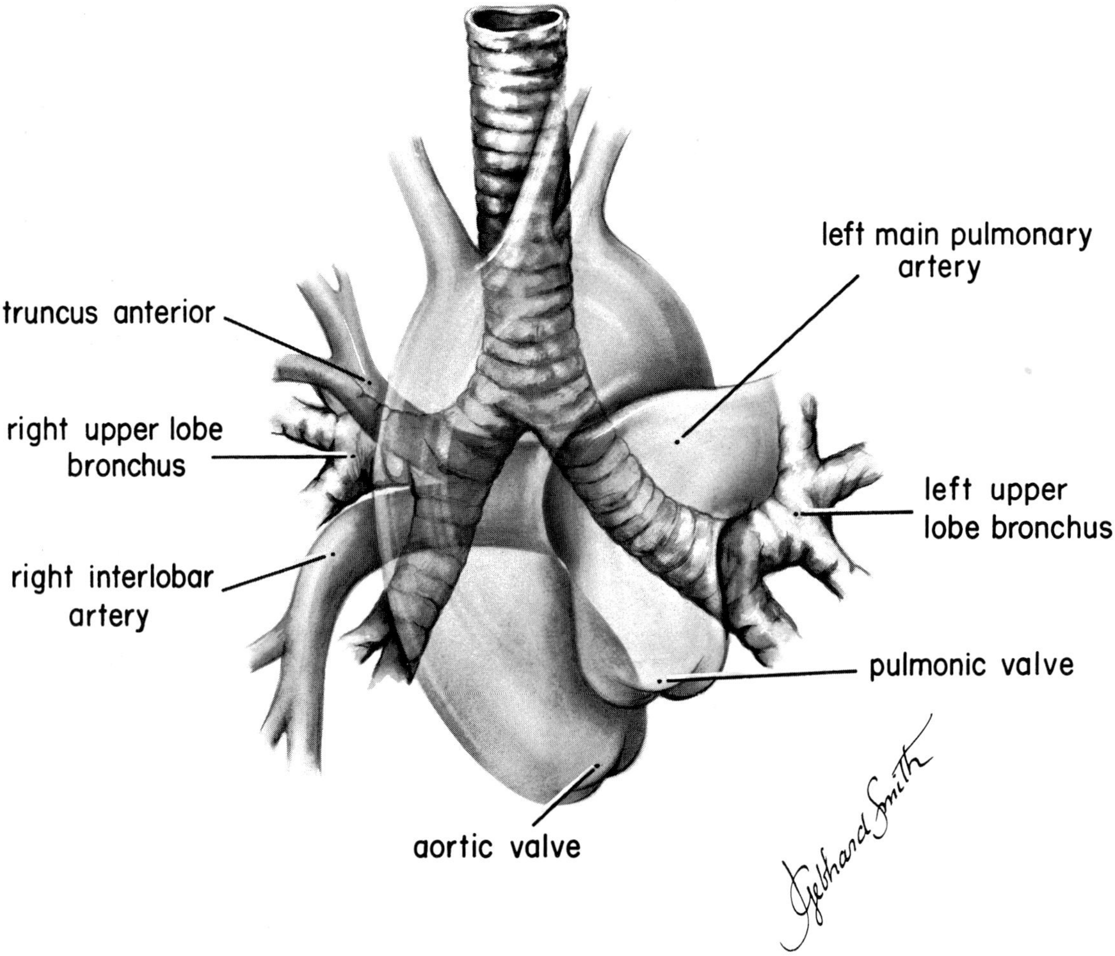

Figure 1–33. **Anatomic Relationship between the Central Pulmonary Arteries, the Tracheobronchial Tree, and the Aorta.** The *right pulmonary artery* lies posterior to the ascending aorta and anterior to the right main bronchus. Its superior branch (the truncus anterior) curves superiorly and anteriorly over the upper-lobe bronchus; its inferior branch (the interlobar artery) passes in front of the intermediate bronchus and curves abruptly downward along the lateral aspect of this bronchus. The *left pulmonary artery* passes immediately anterior and lateral to the lower portion of the left main bronchus; the lower of its two main branches in the hilum (the interlobar artery) curves slightly posteriorly over the top of the upper-lobe bronchus and descends abruptly along the lateral aspect of the lower-lobe bronchus (*see* Figure 1–38, page 43).

artery) is much larger than the truncus anterior (Figure 1–34); it passes in front of the intermediate bronchus and on the lateral aspect of this bronchus descends abruptly into the major fissure. It supplies one branch (in 50 per cent of cases, two branches) to the middle lobe, one to the superior segment of the lower lobe, and, in random order, four branches which accompany the basal bronchi of the lower lobe. As in the bronchial tree, the anterior basilar artery, which extends into the lateral costophrenic sulcus, is the most laterally situated basilar artery.

The *left pulmonary artery* splits into two branches within the left hilum after passing immediately anterior and lateral to the lower portion of the left main bronchus (Figure 1–34). The left pulmonary artery is on a more posterior plane than the right, a difference which usually allows of distinction between the two vessels on lateral roentgenograms. The upper (and smaller) of the two divisions of the left pulmonary artery sends two or more branches to the apical posterior segments and one to the anterior segment of the upper lobe, following closely the anatomic distribution of the

p.a. CXR angio

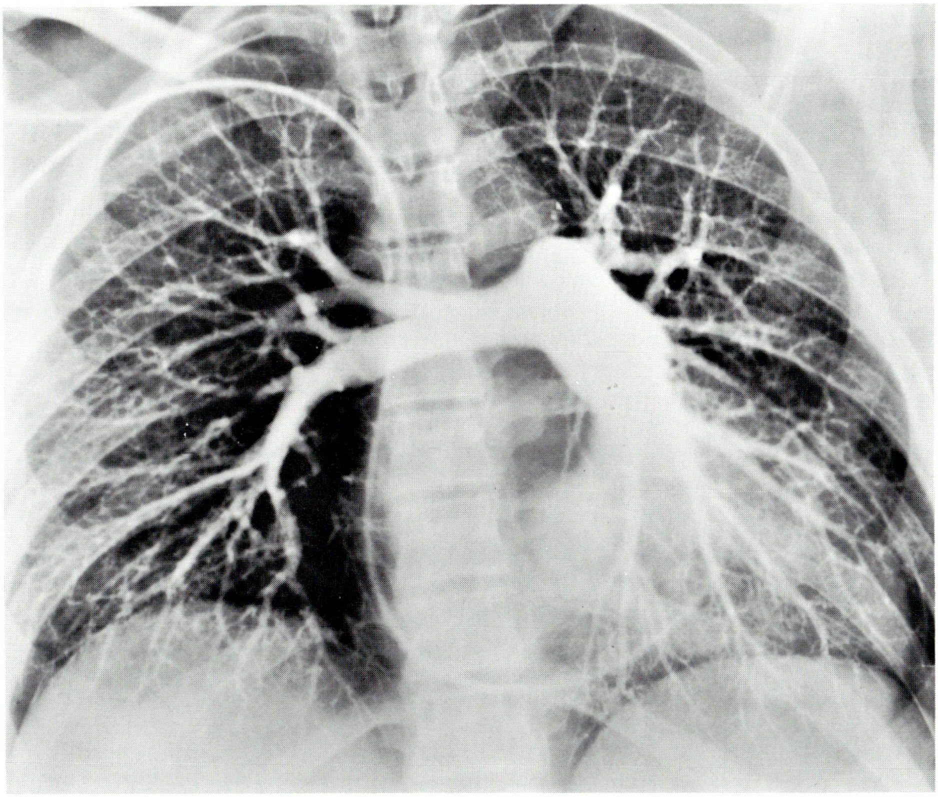

Figure 1–34. **Pulmonary Angiogram.** Arterial phase. *See* text for description.

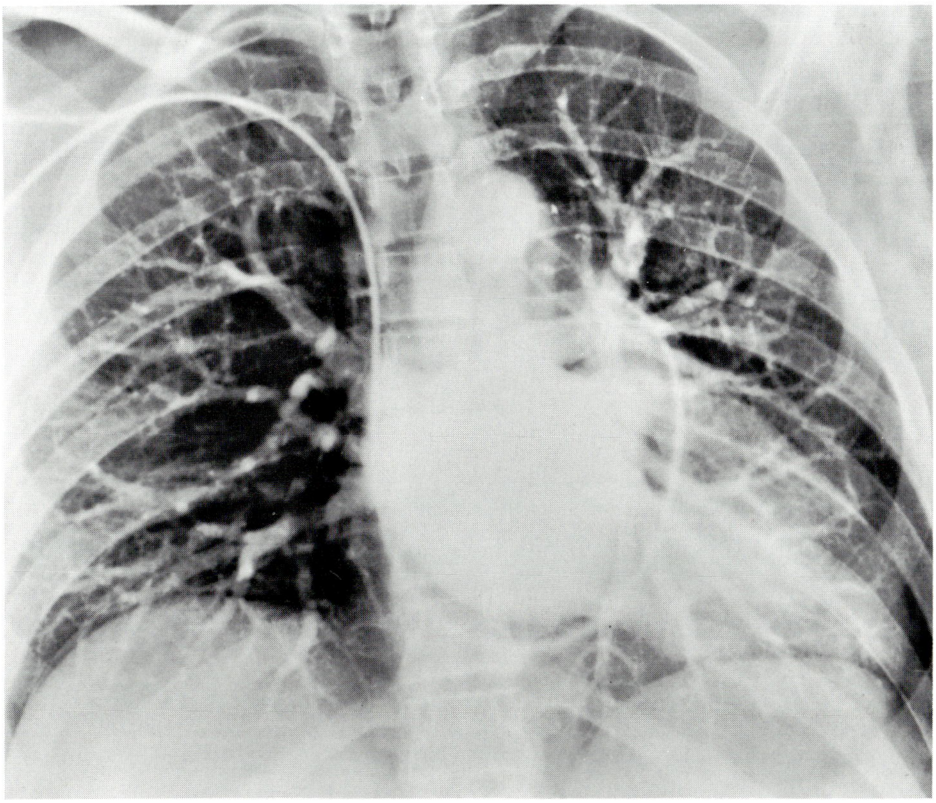

Figure 1–35. **Pulmonary Angiogram.** Venous phase. *See* text for description.

segmental bronchi. Thus, no major vessel to the left upper lobe is analogous to the truncus anterior to the right. The lower of the two main vessels in the hilum (the interlobar artery) curves sharply over the top of the upper-lobe bronchus and descends abruptly, along the lateral aspect of the lower-lobe bronchus, into the major fissure (*see* Figure 1–68, page 94). The lingular artery, with its two branches, arises from the anterior aspect of this vessel. The superior segmental artery of the lower lobe arises from the posterior aspect of the descending artery, just proximal to the origin of the lingular artery. The arterial ramifications to the remainder of the lower lobe are similar in name and number to the basal bronchi they accompany.

The spatial distribution of pulmonary veins is even more variable than that of the arteries (Figures 1–35 and 1–36). The prevailing pattern comprises two large veins on each side which enter the mediastinum at a level slightly below the pulmonary arteries and anterior to them. On the right side, the superior pulmonary veins drain the upper lobe and usually the middle lobe, although in some cases a separate vein from the middle lobe drains directly into the left atrium or joins with the inferior pulmonary vein; the inferior vein drains the whole of the lower lobe. On the left side, the superior and inferior pulmonary veins drain the upper and lower lobes, respectively, although occasionally lingular drainage is into the inferior vein.

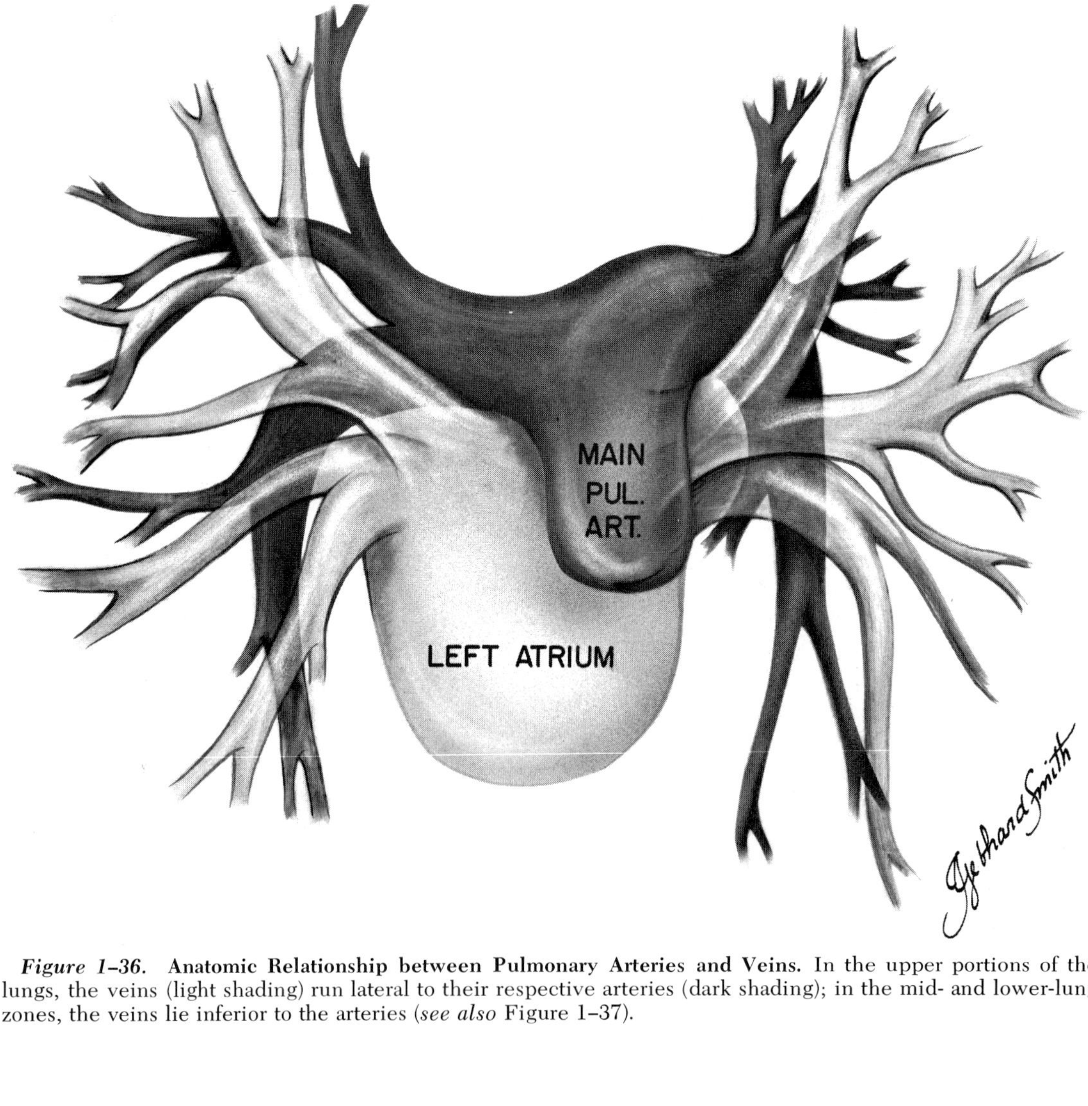

Figure 1–36. **Anatomic Relationship between Pulmonary Arteries and Veins.** In the upper portions of the lungs, the veins (light shading) run lateral to their respective arteries (dark shading); in the mid- and lower-lung zones, the veins lie inferior to the arteries (*see also* Figure 1–37).

Distinction between arterial and venous trunks within the lung fields often can be made without difficulty if certain anatomic relationships are borne in mind (Figure 1–36). The course of the veins within the lungs is remote from the bronchoarterial bundles. This remoteness begins in the periphery of the lungs, where the arterial system is in the center of the lobules and the venous system is within the interlobular septa. This relationship persists, so that in all areas the arteries and their corresponding veins are separated by air-containing lung parenchyma and, thus, should be distinguishable (Figure 1–37). In the upper lobes, the veins run either lateral or inferior to their respective arteries; for example, in the apical segment the vein lies lateral to its artery, whereas in the anterior and posterior segments the relatively horizontal position of the vascular channels is such that the veins lie inferior to the arteries. This inferior relationship of vein to artery usually exists in the right middle lobe and lingula also. Distinction between arteries and veins usually is easier in the lower lobes because of the general vascular topography: the relatively horizontal position of the venous channels contrasts with the almost vertical course of the arteries, a relationship which is particularly well demonstrated in the right lower lobe on a frontal roentgenogram. In the lateral projection, confluence of the pulmonary veins is on a plane slightly anterior to the course of the pulmonary arteries; in this position, the inferior pulmonary vein on the left side often is visualized as a well-circumscribed, round or oval density at its entry into the left atrium—an appearance that should not be mistaken for a mass lesion. As might be expected, throughout the lung fields the caliber and density of the veins are roughly equal to those of their companion arteries.

Although with experience it is often possible to distinguish arteries from veins on standard roentgenograms of the chest in various projections, the confusion of linear shadows may cause some difficulty in identification. The improvement in visualization of vascular shadows to be gained from tomography has been stressed by numerous authors,[71-74] and this technique is strongly recommended when it is important to assess spatial distribution and caliber of the vascular tree (Figure 1–37). In the region of the hila, particularly, tomography may be the only method by which the confusion of vascular shadows may be sorted out; in this situation, the lateral projection often is more revealing than the anteroposterior, as emphasized by Simon[75] (Figure 1–38).

The importance in roentgenographic diagnosis of a proper assessment of the caliber of the hilar pulmonary arteries is considerable. There is little doubt that the most significant sign is a change in the caliber from one examination to another, particularly in relation to the diagnosis of pulmonary embolism; when comparison is not possible or when evidence of pulmonary arterial hypertension is sought, appreciation of the rapidity of tapering of the arteries as they proceed distally is more reliable than mensuration. Roentgenographic measurement of segments of the pulmonary vascular tree appears to us to be of limited value, particularly since it is difficult to establish reproducible reference points for measurement. The figures supplied by Chang,[76] who measured the right descending pulmonary artery in more than 1000 normal adult subjects, appear to be the most accurate available. This author found the normal upper limit of the transverse diameter of the right descending pulmonary artery during inspiration to be 16 mm in males and 15 mm in females; caliber on inspiration was consistently greater than on expiration, the difference varying from 1 to 3 mm.

Perhaps a more useful method of estimating increase or decrease in pulmonary artery caliber is the artery/bronchus index described by Wójtowicz.[74] In a study of 1200 tomograms of 250 normal subjects, this author showed that the ratio of the transverse diameter of a pulmonary artery to that of the bronchus contiguous to it was independent of age, sex, and type of body-build and that it represents a less subjective and more accurate method of assessing disturbances in the pressure and flow in the pulmonary circulation than is possible with direct measurement of the caliber of the artery itself. We have had no experience with this method but think it useful, especially when pulmonary angiography is not feasible. (Examples of the normal mean values of the artery/bronchus indices are 1.30 immediately distal to the take-off of the right upper-lobe bronchus and 1.40 immediately beyond the origin of the left upper-lobe bronchus.)

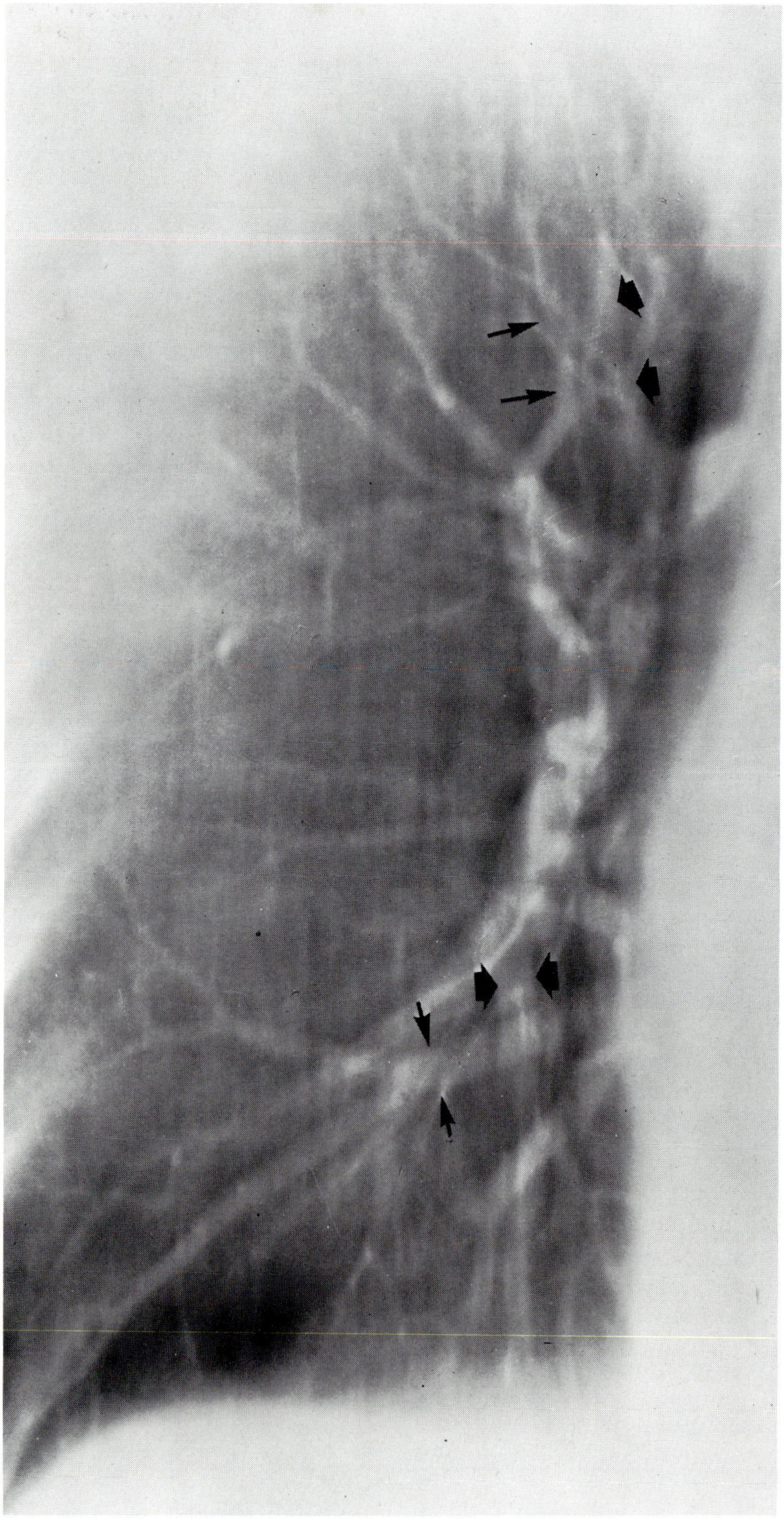

Figure 1–37. **Anatomic Relationship between Pulmonary Arteries and Veins.** Tomographic section of the right lung in AP projection, supine position. Note the lateral relationship of veins (thin arrows) to arteries (thick arrows) in the upper-lung zone. In the lower zone, the relatively horizontal position of the venous channels (thin arrows) contrasts with the almost vertical course of the arteries (thick arrows).

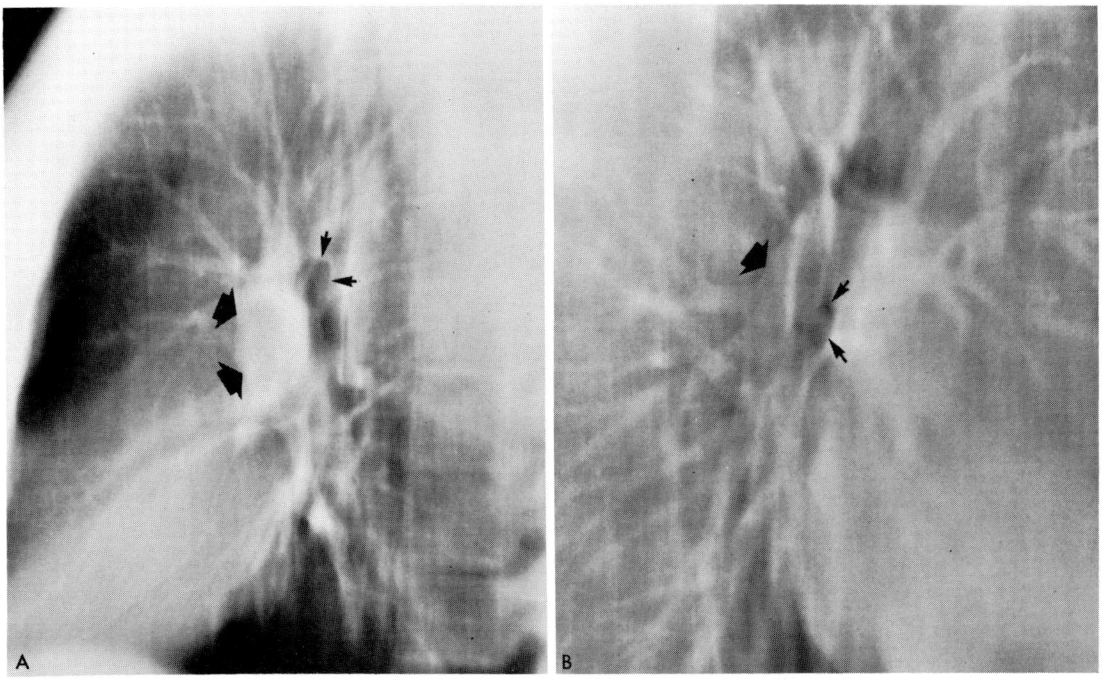

Figure 1–38. **The Hila in Lateral Projection.** *A,* In a lateral tomographic section through the *right* hilum, the tracheal air column is well seen. The oval shadow of the right main pulmonary artery (thick arrows) lies immediately anterior to the air column of the main-stem and intermediate bronchi; immediately above and slightly posterior to this vessel is the circular air column of the right upper-lobe bronchus cut across (thin arrows); the lower-lobe vessels can be seen descending in a slightly posterior direction. *B,* A tomographic section of the *left* hilum reveals certain differences from the right which permits their distinction; the left pulmonary artery is superimposed on the air column of the left main bronchus and immediately above the circular air column of the left upper-lobe bronchus (thin arrows); the interlobar artery (thick arrow) curves posteriorly and inferiorly across the aortic window, giving origin from its posterior surface to the branch of the superior segment of the left lower lobe. The lower-lobe veins can be seen to cross the arteries at a sharp angle.

FUNCTION

Perfusion of the Acinar Unit

Perfusion of acinar units is accomplished through a vast network of thin-walled capillaries which measures 70 to 100 sq m in surface area. The amount of blood in these vessels is estimated to be 60 to 100 ml in the resting subject, increasing to 150 to 250 ml during exercise.[22, 77-80] It is of interest that these figures, which were calculated by measuring uptake of carbon monoxide by red blood cells flowing through capillaries, agree closely with estimates made by anatomic techniques.[81, 82] This may be interpreted as indicating that the capillary vascular bed is maximally distended during peak exercise.[80]

Various pressures modify the flow of blood through the capillaries. (1) *The intravascular pressure* has a mean value of only 14 mm Hg in the pulmonary artery, despite the fact that it handles the same cardiac output as the systemic circulation. (2) *The transmural vascular pressure* is the intravascular pressure minus intrapleural pressure in larger vessels lying outside the lobular limiting membrane. In smaller vessels and capillaries lying within the membrane it is best expressed as the difference between intravascular hydrostatic pressure and alveolar pressure. (3) *The driving pressure* in the pulmonary circulation is the difference between arterial and pulmonary venous or left atrial pressures in the lower part of the lung and the difference between arterial and alveolar pressures in the upper part of the lung, in upright subjects at rest (Figure 1–39). The pressure in capillaries cannot be measured directly; it must be more than 5 mm Hg (left atrial pressure) for blood to move, and has been estimated to be about 9 mm Hg

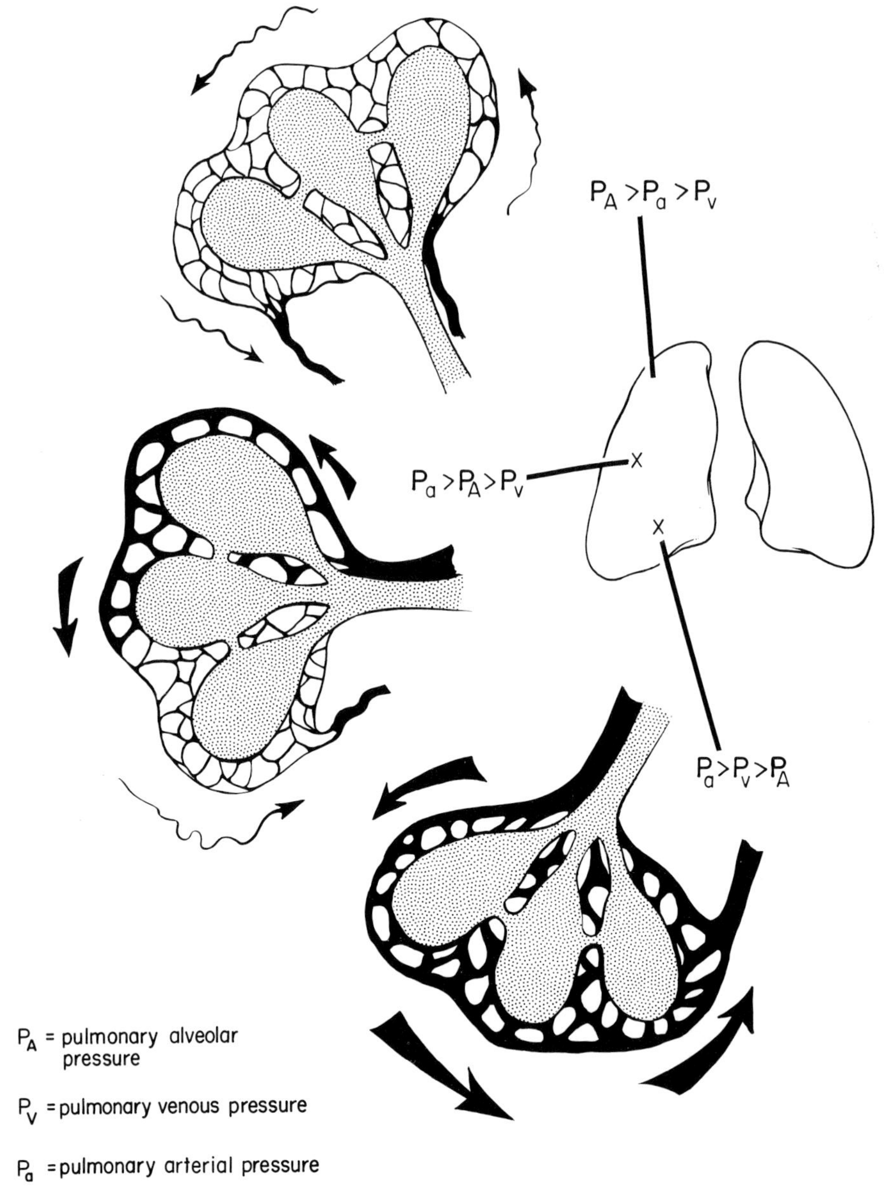

Figure 1–39. **Diagram Depicting the Influence of Gravity on Perfusion of Acinar Units in Upright Man.** *In the upper unit,* alveolar pressure (P_A) is higher than pulmonary artery pressure (P_a) so that the capillaries are virtually empty. *In the mid lung,* alveolar pressure (P_A) is lower than arterial pressure (P_a) but higher than venous pressure (P_v) so that blood flow occurs through the arterial end of the capillaries but is impeded on the venous end. *The unit at the base of the lung* shows dilated capillaries throughout since both arterial (P_a) and venous (P_v) pressures are greater than alveolar pressure (P_A).

at the arterial end and 6 mm Hg at the venous end. Since the colloidal osmotic pressure is thought to be 25 to 30 mm Hg, under normal resting conditions a considerable force keeps the alveoli dry; and even during maximal exercise, when the cardiac output increases to 25 to 30 liters/min, in a healthy man, the hydrostatic pressure does not exceed osmotic pressure.

The hemodynamics of the pulmonary circulation cannot be deduced on the basis of laws that relate to a rigid tubular system. Like the conducting system, the circulatory system is distensible; it branches and bends; it is subject to changing pressure on its walls and has a pressure at each end, either or both of which may vary in degree in certain circumstances. Flow is pulsatile but probably always laminar in small vessels and sometimes turbulent in larger ones. Viscosity is greater in the main vessels, but overall resistance to flow is mainly from arterioles and capillaries. When the left atrial pressure and transpleural (alveolar minus intrapleural) pressure are constant, an increase in pulmonary artery pressure causes vessels to distend (transmural pressure increase). As with the conducting system, doubling or halving the radius causes a 16-fold change in resistance; in this case, as cardiac output increases, vessels widen, and closed capillaries open, leading to a fall in resistance.[83]

SUMMARY. Both physiologic and anatomic measurements indicate that the amount of blood in the capillaries in a resting subject is 60 to 100 ml, increasing to 150 to 250 ml during exercise.

Various pressures influence the flow of blood through pulmonary capillaries. The hydrostatic intravascular pressure in the pulmonary artery has a mean value of only 14 mm Hg. The transmural vascular pressure is the intravascular pressure minus the intrapleural pressure in the larger vessels, and in smaller vessels and capillaries it is believed to be the difference between the intravascular hydrostatic and alveolar pressures. The driving pressure in the pulmonary circulation is greatly influenced by gravity. In erect subjects the driving pressure in the upper lung, where alveolar pressure is greater than pulmonary venous pressure, is the difference between arterial and alveolar pressures. In the lower lung the driving pressure is the difference between arterial and venous pressures.

The intravascular pressure in the capillaries is considered to be in the range of 6 to 9 mm Hg, and the great distensibility of these vessels prevents a significant rise even during severe exertion. The colloidal osmotic pressure is 25 to 30 mm Hg, which serves to keep the alveoli dry even with a five-fold increase in cardiac output.

Factors Which Influence Pulmonary Circulation

GRAVITY. The lung measures approximately 30 cm from apex to base, and the hilum is positioned at about the midline. The pulmonary artery enters the lung at the hilum. Since a column of blood 15 cm high is equivalent to a column of mercury 11 mm high, in the erect subject gravity affects the intravascular pressure to the extent that systolic, diastolic, and mean pressures are reduced by 11 mm Hg at the apex and are increased by 11 mm Hg at the base. If pulmonary arterial pressure in the hilar vessels is taken as 20/9 mm Hg, it follows that pressure at the extreme apex will be 9/ −2, and that no perfusion will occur in the apical zone during diastole; at the base, the pressure will be 31/20, which will cause increase in the capillary pressure in this area and will render the lung base more susceptible to transudation of fluid into the alveoli. Since the pulmonary veins enter the left atrium at approximately the same level, there will be a similar and proportional variation in venous pressure also (Figure 1–39).

The effect of gravity largely governs the distribution of blood flow in the lungs. At the extreme apex in upright man at rest there is no flow simply because the pulmonary arterial pressure is insufficient to overcome the effect of gravity. Farther down the lung, pressure on the arterial side rises but is opposed by alveolar pressure, which readily compresses the thin-walled capillaries. Therefore, the driving pressure in the upper part of the lung is the difference between arterial and alveolar pressures. Since alveolar pressure is not influenced by gravity, and arterial pressure gradually increases down the lung, the driving pressure and, therefore, blood flow also increase. However, because intravascular pressure decreases in the passage of blood from arteriole to venule, alveolar pressure is greater than venous pressure in the upper lung, and the venous end of the capillary is constricted; the degree of constriction decreases gradually as the increasing effect of gravity causes a rise in venous pressure and allows a greater flow of blood as the lung base is approached (Figure 1–39). At one point, venous pressure rises above alveolar pressure, and below that point the driving pressure of blood through the lung is the difference between arterial and venous pressures. Despite the fact that the driving pressure does not increase, because arterial and venous pressures are influenced equally by gravity, blood flow continues to increase as the base of the lung is approached; this is due to the increasing intravascular pressure or transmural pressure on both arterial and venous ends, which dilates the vessels and thereby reduces pulmonary vascular resistance to flow.

Summary. The effect of gravity is to reduce the pulmonary circulation in the upper lung and to increase it in the lower lung. There is no circulation in the capillaries at the extreme apex in erect resting subjects. The pulmonary artery pressure increases from apex to base, and circulation in the capillaries occurs as soon as the pulmonary intravascular pressure is greater than the alveolar pressure. The driving pressure of blood through the lungs becomes the difference between arterial and venous pressures as soon as the effect of gravity causes the pulmonary venous pressure to exceed the alveolar pressure. As the base of the lung is approached, pulmonary circulation continues to increase, not because of an increase in driving pressure—which cannot occur, because arterial and venous pressures are equally affected by gravity—but through the increased transmural pressure, which dilates the pulmonary vasculature and reduces resistance.

INTRAPLEURAL PRESSURE AND LUNG VOLUME. We have seen that the conducting system to the acinar unit runs in two separate "lung compartments." Similarly, larger arteries and veins are outside the lobular limiting membrane and are influenced by their own transmural pressures, the vessels dilating during inspiration as the pressure difference between the lumen and intrapleural "spaces" increases and constricting during expiration as the pressure difference decreases. Vessels within the limiting membrane, like the membranous airways, are affected by changes in lung volume. The small muscular arteries and arterioles lie beside the airways, whereas the veins are between the lobules at the periphery. During inspiration, the increase in lung volume results in dilatation of the vessels, which are closely interconnected with alveolar tissue within the compartment. During expiration, as the lung assumes a position of rest, the vessels narrow and their blood volume decreases.

It is not known what effect changes in lung volume exert on the pulmonary capillaries. Some believe that dilatation of the capillaries causes pulmonary vascular resistance to decrease during lung inflation.[84] The majority, however, consider that these thin-walled vessels are compressed during inspiration, with a resultant increase in vascular resistance.[85-87] There is reason to believe that the compression of the pulmonary capillary bed, with its consequent decrease in blood volume, is offset by the rise in volume in the larger vessels during inspiration.[88] Still an unknown quantity in this regard is the part played by surface tension, which is thought to increase as alveoli distend (*see* page 34) and, consequently, would be expected to counteract the effect of compression by pulling away from capillary walls. This concept is not supported by studies of quickly frozen, living lung tissues, which show the alveolus not as a globular or hemispherical structure but as a polygonal figure with mostly flat septa. However, the possibility remains that surface tension of considerable degree exerts an influence on the vessels at the angles of the septa, where curvature is pronounced.[22, 89]

SUMMARY. The larger pulmonary arteries and veins dilate during inspiration as the difference between intravascular and intrapleural pressures (transmural pressure) increases and constrict during expiration as the pressure difference decreases. The smaller arteries and arterioles, closely interconnected with alveolar tissue, dilate as lung volume increases during inspiration and narrow during expiration. The capillaries probably are compressed during inspiration, leading to an increase in resistance. Surface tension in the alveoli, which increases during inspiration, may counteract the compressing effect of alveolar distention.

NEUROGENIC AND CHEMICAL EFFECTS. In addition to the pressure and volume changes which passively influence the pulmonary vasculature, some active stimuli can modify capillary circulation to acinar units. Hypoxemia and acidosis appear to be the most potent of these. Such stimuli have not only a vasomotor effect but also a direct action on the myocardium (and, hence, on cardiac output) as well as an indirect effect on both myocardium and vessels via the sympathicoadrenal system; thus, their influence on the hemodynamics of the pulmonary circulation is complex.[90] Systemic hypoxemia acts on the carotid body and triggers a reflex mechanism that gives rise to arteriolar vasoconstriction. Local hypoxia is reported to produce vasoconstriction locally,[91] probably by acting on the arteriole that accompanies the terminal bronchiole, *i.e.*, in the circulation which supplies the acinar unit—an ideal area in which to reduce circulation when ventilation is inadequate.[92] Acidosis, whether metabolic (diabetic ketosis, renal failure, or lactic acidosis) or resulting from an increase in the P_{CO_2}, also causes local vasoconstriction and in poorly ventilated acini acts synergistically with the hypoxemic effect. An increased left atrial or pulmonary venous pressure is thought to be the stimulus for production of arteriolar constriction, which protects capillaries from excessive hydrostatic pressure in such conditions as mitral stenosis.[93, 94, 198]

Both the arterial and the venous circulation are sensitive to various drugs (*e.g.*, epinephrine, isoproterenol, serotonin, and histamine) under experimental conditions, but the significance of these findings in relation to the human lung in health or in disease is not known.

The effects of precapillary and postcapillary hypertension on pulmonary hemodynamics are considered in more detail in later sections in relation to the diseases which produce these conditions. The existence of precapillary anastomotic channels between bronchial and pulmonary vessels in the normal lung is controversial, but it is known that they are present in certain disease states. Several types have been found in association with congenital pulmonary artery stenosis, bronchiectasis, and pulmonary diseases that give rise to interstitial fibrosis,[68] and their functioning has been demonstrated by use of angiographic techniques and by analysis of oxygen saturation during catheterization of lobar arteries.[95, 179] Since systemic arterial pressure is six to eight times greater than pulmonary artery pressure, flow is from bronchial to pulmonary vessels; as Liebow[96] has pointed out, vascular resistance is increased in these diseased areas, thus allowing blood in the pulmonary circulation to be diverted to better functioning lung units.

SUMMARY. Hypoxemia and acidosis appear to be potent vasomotor stimuli to the pulmonary vasculature. A local vasoconstrictive effect, possibly at the level of the arteriole accompanying the terminal bronchiole, is considered to be responsible for preventing circulation of poorly ventilated acinar units. In certain disease states, bronchial—pulmonary artery anastomoses may increase the vascular resistance in damaged and underventilated areas, thereby diverting pulmonary blood flow to functioning units.

Diffusion of Gas from Acinar Units to Red Blood Cells

DIFFUSION IN THE ACINAR UNIT. Diffusion of a gas occurs passively from an area of higher partial pressure of the gas to one of lower partial pressure. In a gaseous medium, a light gas diffuses faster than a heavier one. In a liquid or in tissue the rate of diffusion is largely dependent upon the solubility of the particular gas in that medium. Oxygen is slightly lighter than carbon dioxide and, therefore, diffuses more rapidly in acinar gas. In water and tissue, carbon dioxide is more soluble than oxygen, and diffuses through these media 20 times faster than does oxygen. Since both are able to diffuse many thousands of times more rapidly in a gaseous medium than in water or tissue, diffusion out of acini consists largely in getting through the alveolocapillary membrane and plasma and in and out of the red cell. Because diffusion through these structures is accomplished much more readily by carbon dioxide than by oxygen, outward diffusion of carbon dioxide never is a clinical problem, and further discussion need concern only the diffusion of oxygen.

Assuming a tidal volume of 450 ml and a dead space of 150 ml, 300 ml of fresh air and 150 ml of dead-space alveolar air from the previous expiration enters the acinar units during each inspiration (Figure 1–29, page 31). Since the units already contain seven or eight times this volume (functional residual capacity), the "fresh" air which enters last may fill only the respiratory bronchioles and main ducts. In the normal lung, however, because of the rapid diffusion of oxygen in a gaseous medium, complete mixing of this fresh air with intra-acinar gas is probably instantaneous. In obstructive emphysema, with the breakdown of alveolar septa and the creation of much larger air spaces, mixing may be delayed, and in these circumstances gaseous diffusion may limit the diffusing capacity.[199]

DIFFUSION ACROSS THE ALVEOLOCAPILLARY MEMBRANE. The membrane through which oxygen diffuses to reach plasma in capillaries comprises (1) a surface-active liquid which lines the intra-alveolar membrane, (2) alveolar epithelial cells with attenuated cytoplasm, (3) basement membrane to the epithelial layer, (4) loose connective tissue, (5) basement membrane to the capillary endothelium, and (6) capillary endothelium. Schulz[97] considers that diffusion takes place only through the lateral cytoplasmic extensions of the alveolar epithelial cells, and states that the "blood-air pathway" in a normal lung is 0.36 to 2.5μ thick. Through this thin membrane, with a driving pressure of approximately 60 mm Hg (Po_2 of alveolar gas minus Po_2 of mixed venous blood [$100 - 40 = 60$ mm Hg]), under resting conditions oxygen almost fully saturates the blood in one-third of the time taken by blood to traverse the pulmonary capillaries. During exercise, with increased cardiac output and pulmonary capillary blood volume, the transit time is reduced: nevertheless, aided by the slightly higher Po_2 due to increased ventilation, the blood is virtually saturated by oxygen by the time it reaches the end of the capillary. With decreased alveolar Po_2 (*e.g.*, due to atmospheric conditions at high altitude, respiratory-center depression, or neuromuscular disease), the driving pressure of oxygen is reduced; exercise under these conditions results in a shortened transit time which, together with the reduced driving pressure, may limit diffusion, so that the end-capillary blood may be only partly oxygenated. Although the transit time is thought of in relation to capillaries only, it is probable that the process of diffusion starts in the arterioles which are the origin of capillaries, since their walls are in direct contact with alveolar air.[22, 24, 171]

In addition to the aforementioned factors which affect diffusion, the total area in which flowing blood comes in contact with ventilated acinar units influences the capacity for diffusion. This is exemplified by the decrease in diffusion which occurs after pneumonectomy[1] and may be responsible in part for the decrease in diffusing capacity which occurs in emphysema—in which disease a considerable amount of the alveolocapillary membrane often is destroyed. The amount of *effective* alveolocapillary membrane often is reduced because of mismatching of capillary circulation with acinar ventilation (*see* page 52); since this may be an inevitable accompaniment of diseases which cause thickening of the alveolocapillary membrane, assessment of responsibility for diffusion impairment may be difficult.[98, 99]

Many diseases may involve the acinar unit in such a way as to interfere with diffusion (Figure 1–40). In such cases the arterial oxygen saturation may be normal in patients at rest, despite significant reduction in diffusing capacity; however, exercise elicits hypoxemia because the transit time through capillaries is decreased.

INTRAVASCULAR DIFFUSION. The crossing of the alveolocapillary membrane by oxygen does not complete the process of diffusion, and it is probable that resistance to gas movement into red cells often is greater than that to gas movement from the alveoli into the blood.[100] This is due not to the distance to be traversed through plasma to the red cell but to the rate of reaction of oxygen molecules with red-cell contents. Differences in the rate of gas exchange in the red cell, the final phase of diffusion, are not important in relation to normal lungs breathing air, but they play a significant role in diffusion impairment in states of low alveolar oxygen tension and in anemia.

MEASUREMENT OF DIFFUSING CAPACITY. Measurement of the capacity for diffusion of oxygen is a very complicated and perhaps unreliable procedure. It is necessary to know the mixed venous Po_2, in order to determine the driving pressure of oxygen; and the rate of diffusion varies along the capillary as the driving pressure decreases while the Po_2 in capillary blood increases. Because of these problems, carbon monoxide generally is used to measure diffusion; it has a great affinity for hemoglobin and, therefore, only a minute quantity of a low concentration (0.3 per cent) is required. The diffusing capacity for carbon monoxide is the amount of this gas taken up per minute, divided by the difference between partial pressures of carbon monoxide in the alveolus and in capillary blood. Since there is no carbon monoxide in mixed venous blood, the amount of gas taken up is the difference between the carbon monoxide content of inspired and expired gas. The denominator of the equation is equal to the mean alveolar Pco_2, which can be calculated from an end-tidal sample; the mean capillary Pco_2 is so small that it can be ignored. Several techniques have been developed for using this gas; the advantages of particular methods were discussed in detail by Bates and Christie.[1]

SUMMARY. The diffusion of oxygen from alveolus to red blood cell is influenced by the difference between alveolar and mixed venous P_{O_2}, the total area and thickness of alveolocapillary membrane, and the number of red blood cells and their transit time in the pulmonary capillaries. For technical reasons the diffusing capacity is measured most conveniently and accurately with minute quantities of a low concentration of carbon monoxide.

The Matching of Capillary Blood Flow with Ventilation in the Acinus

Ideally, alveolar ventilation and alveolar perfusion should be uniform; *i.e.*, each acinus should receive just the right amount of air to oxygenate the hemoglobin completely and to remove the carbon dioxide

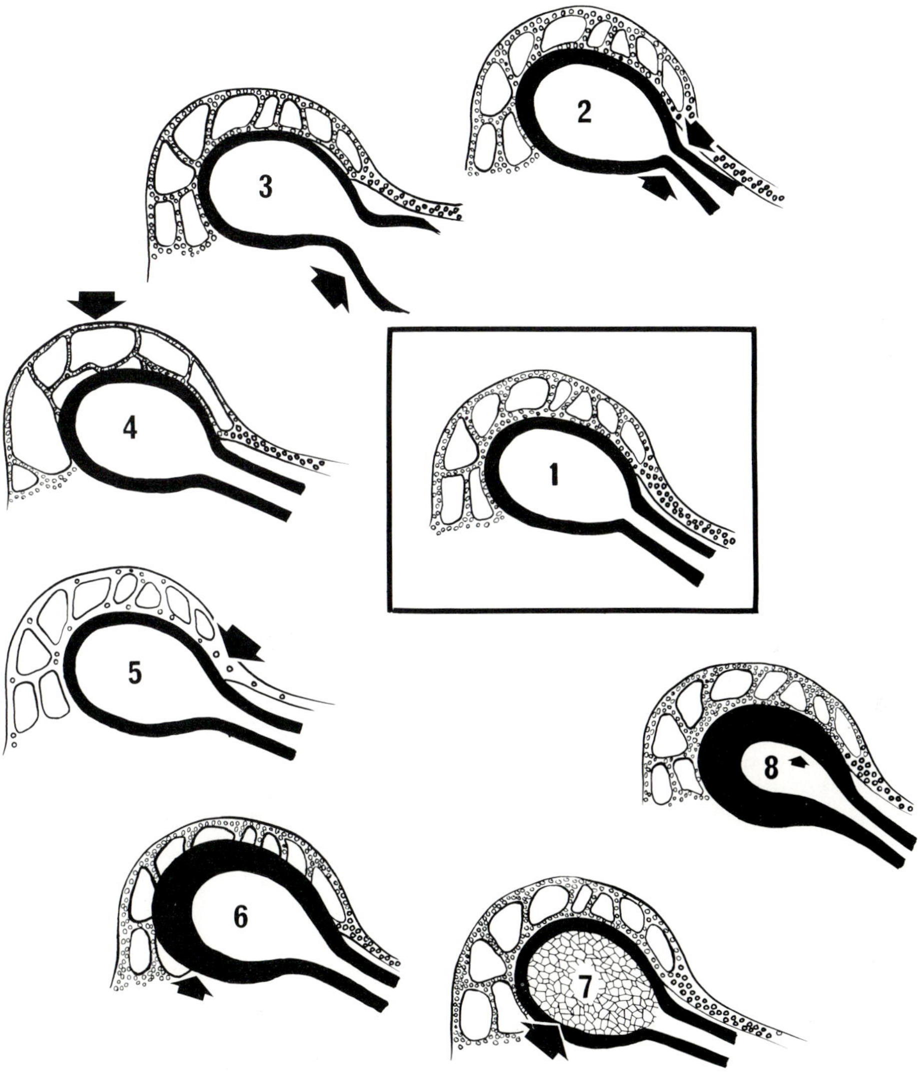

Figure 1–40. **Pathophysiology of Diffusion Defect.** The structure in the center of the diagram (1) is a normal air-containing acinar unit in which are depicted a conducting system, an alveolar cell lining, a normal amount of tissue between air space and capillary endothelium, and a capillary network containing a normal number of red blood cells. The acinar units around the periphery depict various mechanisms of diffusion defect:

(2) Obstruction to air entry.
(3) Dilatation and confluence of respiratory bronchioles (resulting in an increased pathway for diffusion, as in centrilobular emphysema).
(4) Loss of capillaries.
(5) Anemia.
(6) Increase in tissue between air space and capillary endothelium.
(7) Replacement of air in air space by edema, exudate, or blood.
(8) Increase in alveolar lining cells.

given off during gas exchange. This would mean that each of the 33,000 acini, with its 400 alveolar ducts and 8000 alveoli, would receive equal portions of the alveolar ventilation ($\dot{V}_A$), which is estimated to average 4.5 liters/min, and of the alveolar perfusion ($\dot{Q}$), which averages 5 liters/min. In other words, not only would the ratio of ventilation to perfusion ($\dot{V}_A/\dot{Q}$) be 4.5:5.0 liters, or 0.9 for each lung, but each acinar unit would have an identical ratio. Despite the fact that this is not true even for the normal lung, the concept of an "ideal" $\dot{V}_A/\dot{Q}$ ratio is useful as a point of reference in judging relationships between ventilation and perfusion within the acini.

When the $\dot{V}_A/\dot{Q}$ ratio is not ideal, *i.e.*, other than 0.9, it is either because perfusion is reduced relative to ventilation or because ventilation is decreased relative to blood flow.

The effect of gravity is to increase blood flow to the most dependent portion of lung. In upright man this is the lung base. As stated (*see* page 45), the increase in blood flow in the middle part of the lung is due to a rising hydrostatic pressure in the arteries and arterioles; since intra-alveolar pressure does not change, the rise in hydrostatic pressure causes an increase in driving pressure. In the lower lung, where pulmonary venous pressure exceeds alveolar, the driving pressure of blood through the lung is the difference between pressure on the arterial end and that on the venous end of the capillary. Since gravity affects the intravascular pressure on the venous end to the same extent as on the arterial end, the driving pressure does not change as the base of the lung is approached. However, vessel distention caused by the increase in intramural pressure reduces resistance in this part of the pulmonary circulation and thus permits ever-increasing blood flow down to the lung base.

Ventilation of the lung is modified by gravity also.[101] The effect of gravity is to increase intrapleural pressure down the lung, *i.e.*, make it less subatmospheric, and thus decrease transpulmonary pressure. Therefore, at the end of a quiet expiration, the acinar units are less distended and their volume is smaller in the lower than in the upper lung regions. During the next inspiration, any change in transpulmonary pressure results in relatively more regional ventilation of lower than of upper lung zones. In other words, since functional residual capacity is proportionally less in lower than in upper lung regions, the lower regions receive a larger percentage of inspired air. If this increase in ventilation from apex to base were directly proportional to the increase in blood flow, the $\dot{V}_A/\dot{Q}$ ratio would not vary throughout the lung. However, this is not the case, and since the effect of gravity is greater on perfusion than on ventilation, blood and gas are slightly mismatched; *i.e.*, the $\dot{V}_A/\dot{Q}$ ratio changes down the lung.

For many years various methods which use inert gases, such as helium, nitrogen, and argon, have been used to determine the distribution of inspired gas to the alveoli. There tests detect the presence of poorly ventilated areas but do not locate them and yield normal values when ventilation is uniform, even when perfusion is uneven.

Areas with reduced and absent perfusion contribute little or no carbon dioxide to the expired air; if their volume of ventilation is large enough they cause significant dilution of the carbon dioxide to the total expired gas, since inspired gas going to unperfused areas contains insignificant amounts of carbon dioxide and the gas is expired virtually unchanged. In such circumstances, comparison of the P_{CO_2} of arterial blood and that of expired gas coming from the alveoli shows that the normal gradient of 2 mm Hg is increased to 6 mm Hg, or more. As with methods using inert gases for the detection of abnormal distribution of ventilation, this demonstration of abnormal distribution of perfusion indicates only that this mismatching of blood and gas exists and does not locate it.

More recently, radioactive gases have been used to determine regional ventilation and perfusion.[102-104] These techniques detect the presence of inequality of perfusion and ventilation at various levels in the lungs of normal subjects. The counters, which measure the radioactivity, "look" at many hundreds of acinar units at one time and obviously reflect the sum total of their $\dot{V}_A/\dot{Q}$ ratios. In contrast to other methods of assessing ventilation and perfusion distribution, they record the ratios which obtain regionally. These methods are useful in studies of the normal lung and are proving their worth in measurement of lung function in various diseases.[105, 106]

At least three groups using radioactive gases have shown beyond question that gravity changes the $\dot{V}_A/\dot{Q}$ ratio from "ideal" values in the normal subject.[102-104] The $\dot{V}_A/\dot{Q}$ ratio varies between 2 and 3 at the apex of the lung and between 0.5 and 1.0 at the base. The top-to-bottom gravity effect is absent when the subject is supine and is reversed in the head-down position; it is exaggerated at the apices when pulmonary arterial pressure falls and at both top and bottom during acceleration of the body. This last maneuver not only deprives the upper lung of blood but also diverts flow to the lower lung, which may be unventilated because of closure of the conducting system due to the increase in intrapleural pressure.[107]

INCREASED VENTILATION/PERFUSION RATIOS. Increase in the $\dot{V}_A/\dot{Q}$ ratio indicates too much ventilation in relation to the amount of blood flowing through that area. Under normal conditions the highest ratios are at the extreme apices of the lungs, where it is believed there are acini which are not perfused in man standing at rest. Therefore, the ratio in such an acinus which is still ventilated can be expressed as infinity. The existence of such units is predicted from knowledge of the effect of gravity on intravascular pressure, which indicates that alveolar pressure is higher than capillary in this region. There is some evidence, however, that perfusion of the lung occurs even when capillary pressure is slightly less than alveolar pressure;[108, 109] intra-alveolar surface tension, pulling away from the capillary wall and thus keeping the capillary open, has been credited with responsibility for this phenomenon,[108] but results of Staub's studies of frozen lung tissue do not support this explanation.[22]

Ventilation of totally underperfused acinar units serves no purpose; neither does a portion of that to units which are overventilated relative to their perfusion. It is possible to determine the disproportion in ventilation in relation to blood flow; this volume is referred to as "wasted ventilation" or "alveolar dead space." When it is added to the volume of the conducting system, *i.e.*, the anatomic dead space, the total is expressed as the "physiologic" dead space. This may be greatly increased in certain disease states, such as embolism to large pulmonary arteries, in which ventilation persists despite little or no circulation, or when large bullous or cystic areas communicate with the conducting system. In such conditions a decreased number of acinar units is available for gas exchange, and, if cardiac output remains unchanged, it follows that ventilation has to increase to expel the usual amount of carbon dioxide and to maintain the usual level of oxygenation. The P_{CO_2} of arterial blood can be kept within normal limits by this adjustment (*see* page 52), but the P_{CO_2} of the end-tidal gas (the expired gas, after subtracting the volume from the anatomic dead space) is reduced because of the contribution from the alveolar dead space. This alveolar-arterial gradient for P_{CO_2} can result only from overventilation relative to perfusion, *i.e.*, a predominance of acinar units with high $\dot{V}_A/\dot{Q}$ ratios.

DECREASED VENTILATION/PERFUSION RATIOS. Conversely—and this applies to the base of the lung in normal upright man—there may be too little ventilation in relation to the amount of pulmonary blood flow. In such circumstances, an acinar unit, which is totally unventilated but is perfused, has a $\dot{V}_A/\dot{Q}$ ratio of zero. An underventilated unit does not raise the P_{O_2} or lower the P_{CO_2} of the end-capillary blood to the same degree as does a unit with uniform ventilation and perfusion. Therefore blood leaving acinar units with low $\dot{V}_A/\dot{Q}$ ratios and going to the left side of the heart and to the systemic circulation decreases the P_{O_2} of arterial blood and increases the P_{CO_2}. This is equivalent to saying that there is some "wasted blood flow" from these units, analogous to the wasted ventilation, which contributes to the expired gas from units that are overventilated relative to their blood flow. This blood adds to the venous admixture caused by "absolute shunts," which exist even in normal lungs. Absolute shunting, *i.e.*, the passage of venous blood through the lungs, without any contact with alveolar gas, occurs in the normal state because bronchial blood flow is partially taken up in the pulmonary venules. In diseased lungs, absolute shunts may develop between pulmonary arterioles and venules, by-passing acinar units, and may contribute significant amounts of blood to the venous admixture. The relative amounts of blood contributed to the venous admixture by absolute shunts and by acini with low $\dot{V}_A/\dot{Q}$ ratios can be calculated while the subject breathes 100 per cent oxygen.

Poorly ventilated acini may result from a loss of distensibility (compliance) of the lung units, from the presence of obstruction to flow (resistance) in the conducting system, which prevents satisfactory ventilation in the time taken for a respiratory cycle, or from an abnormally long distance for gas diffusion to the alveolar wall. Regardless of cause, the inhalation of 100 per cent oxygen results in gradual replacement of nitrogen by oxygen, even in the most poorly ventilated unit, so that blood leaving the unit becomes fully saturated. On the other hand, this inspired gas with a high Po_2 (670 mm Hg) does not come in contact with blood flowing through absolute shunts. It follows that any hypoxemia of arterial blood that remains during the inspiration of 100 per cent oxygen is due to absolute shunting. However, because 100 per cent oxygen not only saturates hemoglobin completely but also dissolves 2 ml oxygen per 100 ml blood, as against 0.3 ml when room air is breathed, an absolute shunt of 20 per cent or less may be undetected if measurement is made of only oxygen saturation of arterial blood and not of Po_2. This is because oxygen dissolved in plasma attaches to and fully saturates hemoglobin when blood coming from the lungs, which are exposed to a partial pressure of 100 per cent oxygen, mixes with shunted blood on the left side of the heart. The venous admixture from a shunt of 20 per cent or less can be detected, however, by determining the Po_2 of arterial blood—which, in the absence of an absolute shunt, should be approximately 600 mm Hg.

Since both a lowered Po_2 (indirectly) and a raised Pco_2 (directly) stimulate the respiratory center and augment ventilation, it follows that, if some acinar units are underventilated and thus create hypoxemia and hypercarbia, total alveolar ventilation is increased. This affects well-ventilated acinar units in that carbon dioxide is washed out and their alveolar Pco_2 is reduced, which allows for a higher Pco_2 gradient and, therefore, a greater driving pressure for diffusion between blood and gas. Consequently, excess carbon dioxide retained by blood circulating through poorly ventilated units is balanced by an output larger than normal from units that are perfused and well ventilated. Comparison of the dissociation curves for carbon dioxide and oxygen (Figure 1–41) shows that, although this compensation can be readily accomplished for carbon dioxide, the shape of the oxygen curve prevents further significant oxygenation at high levels of Po_2. Even if the ventilation of an acinar unit is doubled, raising the Po_2 from 100 to 125 mm Hg, the curve is so nearly horizontal in this range that arterial oxygen saturation increases from 97.5 per cent to only 98.5 per cent. In other words, ventilation/perfusion inequality leading to hypoxemia is not associated with carbon dioxide retention so long as sufficient numbers of acinar units are well ventilated.

SIGNIFICANCE OF VENTILATION/PERFUSION INEQUALITY. Although gravity effects considerable changes in perfusion and in $\dot{V}A/\dot{Q}$ ratios from top to bottom of the lung, the overall effect on gas exchange in normal upright man is small. It has been estimated that the Po_2 of arterial blood would be only 3 mm Hg higher if perfusion matched ventilation exactly.[107] Increased flow to the lungs, as occurs during exercise or in the presence of left-to-right cardiac shunts, produces a more even distribution of blood, as does pulmonary arterial or venous hypertension.

Unevenness of ventilation and perfusion is the major cause of cyanosis in patients with respiratory disease. However, it is remarkable how severely the lung may be diseased without deviation of the arterial oxygen saturation from the normal range of 95 to 100 per cent: it may remain so when a lobe or even an entire lung has been destroyed by bronchiectasis or emphysema. In many cases this may be explained by the simultaneous destruction by disease of vessels and airways. In such circumstances, despite the fact that both ventilation and perfusion are uneven, they are matched, and the $\dot{V}A/\dot{Q}$ ratios approach "ideal." In addition to these fortuitous "pathologic occurrences," compensatory physiologic mechanisms attempt to maintain $\dot{V}A/\dot{Q}$ ratio and arterial oxygen saturation within normal limits. Since, as pointed out by Staub,[22] the pulmonary microcirculation lacks sphincters and innervation, it appears that blood distribution in capillaries is purely random and is influenced by such minor factors as blocked capillaries (by microembolism and leukocytes) and, perhaps, even the angle of a capillary as it comes off the arteriole. If such is the case, it seems almost essential that some regional

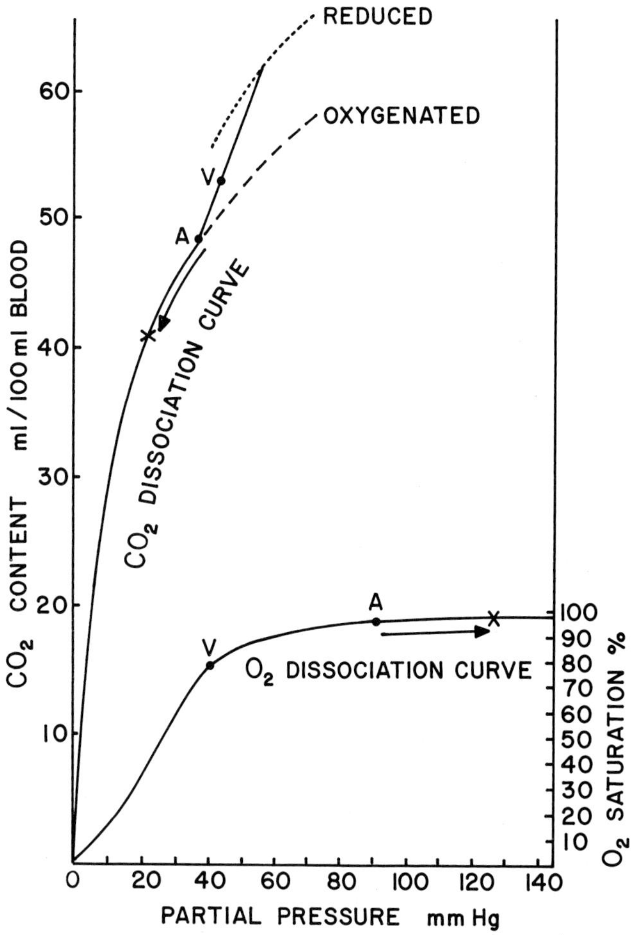

Figure 1–41. **The Carbon Dioxide and Oxygen Dissociation Curves of Blood.** The arrows (A → X) indicate the effect of doubling the ventilation on both CO_2 content and O_2 content (arterial oxygen saturation). The normal values for both arterial (A) and venous (V) oxygen and carbon dioxide are noted. It can be seen that, at any given P_{CO_2}, reduced blood can carry more carbon dioxide than oxygenated blood. *See* text.

control to match ventilation and perfusion should exist at entry to the lung unit. For this reason it seems logical to assume that the very close association of terminal bronchiole and arteriole in the same connective-tissue sheath is more than a chance occurrence. This would be an ideal site to shut off perfusion when ventilation was inadequate or to reduce ventilation when blood flow was lacking. A low P_{O_2} in the gas approaching the acinus may act at this site:[92] by producing a constriction of the pulmonary arteriole it may divert blood to areas which are better ventilated. Studies with an electrode inserted into pulmonary arteries 2 mm in diameter clearly show that inspired gas diffuses into the lumen of such vessels.[171] There is also a mechanism for reducing ventilation in areas with little or no perfusion. The stimulus to this bronchiolar or bronchial constriction is a low P_{CO_2}, but the exact site of action has not been determined.[64, 65, 153]

SUMMARY. Even in the normal lung there is mismatching of ventilation and perfusion. Both are affected by gravity but perfusion to a greater extent than ventilation and, therefore, the upper lung is overventilated and the lower underventilated relative to circulation. The distribution of inspired gas can be detected with the use of inert gases. The distribution of blood can be measured by comparing the P_{CO_2} of arterial blood with the P_{CO_2} of mixed alveolar expired gas. These methods of determining distribution indicate the likelihood of gross mismatching of blood and gas but do not indicate which areas of the lung are responsible. Radioactive gases can be inhaled and can be injected into a systemic vein, and by use of scintillation counters over the chest wall, regional ventilation and perfusion can be estimated. Each counter will measure the sum total of $\dot{V}A/\dot{Q}$ ratios of large numbers of acini.

An *increased* ventilation/perfusion ratio (greater than 0.9) indicates too much ventilation relative to perfusion; such a situation exists normally in the upper lungs. The surplus of ventilation can be calculated and is known as "wasted ventilation." This, together with the anatomic dead space, represents the "physiologic" dead space. In certain disease states, such as pulmonary embolism or large bullae, which communicate with the bronchial tree, the physiologic dead space may be considerable and is reflected in an increase in the arterial–alveolar PCO_2 gradient.

A *decreased* ventilation/perfusion ratio (less than 0.9) indicates too little ventilation relative to perfusion. Such a situation exists normally in the lower lung zones. The surplus of perfusion ("waste blood flow") is indicated by the degree of reduction in arterial blood PO_2.

Hypoxemia due to underventilated alveoli can be distinguished from that due to absolute shunts in the lung when the patient breathes 100 per cent oxygen: this raises the PO_2 to the normal level of 600 mm Hg, or more, in cases of hypoventilation resulting from any cause. Some degree of absolute shunt is present if this level is not reached.

Pulmonary capillary blood leaving underventilated areas is not fully saturated with oxygen and has a raised PCO_2. When there is sufficient healthy lung remaining, an increase in ventilation allows maintenance of the PCO_2 at a normal level in the arterial blood, but, because of the shape of the oxygen-dissociation curve, usually hypoxemia is not corrected.

The effect of gravity in normal upright man is to decrease the PO_2 to 3 mm Hg less than it would be in "ideal" circumstances. Even when the pulmonary parenchyma is largely destroyed there may be very little mismatching of perfusion and ventilation. Simultaneous destruction of circulation and air spaces account for this in part, but there are physiologic mechanisms also which prevent circulation to poorly ventilated areas and ventilation to poorly perfused areas.

Blood Gases and H-ion Concentration (pH)

The ability of the lung to perform its prime function—the exchange of oxygen and carbon dioxide—is readily determined from analysis of a sample of arterial blood. The oxygen carried can be measured as arterial oxygen saturation or as PO_2. Arterial oxygen saturation = O_2 content/O_2 capacity (per cent). Since each 1.0 g of hemoglobin can combine with 1.34 ml O_2, the oxygen capacity of a subject with 15 g hemoglobin per 100 ml blood is approximately 20 ml/100 ml blood. The content is the amount of oxygen that the blood actually contains; this can be determined in a sample by extracting under anaerobic conditions. In a subject with normal lungs breathing air at sea level this amounts to 19 ml (or slightly more) and, therefore, oxygen saturation is $19/20 \times 100$, or 95 per cent.

The PO_2 may be determined from the oxygen-dissociation curve, using arterial oxygen saturation, but this is not truly reliable, because of the almost horizontal slope of the upper part of the curve (*see* Figure 1–41). The PO_2 can be measured directly, by use of an electrode—which, as we have seen, is the only way of determining total oxygen carried by hemoglobin and plasma during the inhalation of 100 per cent oxygen.

In contrast to oxygen, which is carried almost entirely by hemoglobin, approximately 75 per cent of carbon dioxide is contained in plasma. In the resting subject, whereas mixed venous blood holds about 15 ml O_2/100 ml blood at a PO_2 of 40 mm Hg and an oxygen saturation of 75 per cent, its carbon dioxide content is about 52 ml/100 ml blood at a PCO_2 of 45 mm Hg. Although the red blood cell carries only 25 per cent of the carbon dioxide it plays an essential role in the transport of this gas to the lungs; it contains the enzyme carbonic anhydrase, which rapidly hydrates the carbon dioxide passing through the erythrocyte membrane and converts it into carbonic acid, H-ions, and bicarbonate ions. The bicarbonate ions (HCO_3) quickly permeate the cell membrane and enter the plasma in exchange for chloride ions; in this manner, as bicarbonate, most of the carbon dioxide from the tissues is carried by the blood. Since blood which contains reduced hemoglobin can carry more carbon dioxide than can fully oxygenated blood at the same P_{CO_2}, the circumstances are ideal for the uptake of carbon dioxide in the tissues and its unloading in the pulmonary capillaries when the hemoglobin has been reoxygenated (*see* Figure 1–41).

In anemia, no matter how severe, the P_{O_2} is normal and the hemoglobin is fully saturated, oxygen content and capacity being reduced. However, the small amount of oxygen taken up by the blood indicates the presence of the anemia and the resultant reduction in total oxygen transport to the tissues. When normal hemoglobin is replaced by methemoglobin, sulfhemoglobin, or carboxyhemoglobin, the P_{O_2} remains normal, although spectrophotometric analysis of the sample reveals reduction in oxygen saturation.

Arterial hypoxemia may be due to one or more of four mechanisms—diffusion defect, true shunt, ventilation/perfusion inequality, or hypoventilation.

A reduction in diffusing capacity is most commonly seen in emphysema, in which it is due to ventilation/perfusion inequality and loss of alveolocapillary membrane, and in those diseases that give rise to thickening of the alveolocapillary membrane from granulomatous, fibrotic, or neoplastic infiltration. As already mentioned (*see* page 48), this latter group may have $\dot{V}_A/\dot{Q}$ inequality also, which in some undoubtedly plays a major part in reducing the capacity for diffusion. Hypoxemia may be absent at rest, but during exercise, when the intracapillary transit time is reduced, arterial oxygen saturation and P_{O_2} are decreased. The P_{CO_2} is normal or may even be reduced, because carbon dioxide diffuses through a tissue membrane 20 times as readily as oxygen; also, these subjects tend to hyperventilate and thereby produce a decrease in carbon dioxide with a secondary decrease in bicarbonate, to compensate for the respiratory alkalosis.

A true shunt of venous blood to systemic circulation may be due to congenital cardiac disease, arteriovenous aneurysm of the lung, or, in some diseases which affect the parenchyma, precapillary anastomosis of the pulmonary arteriole and venule. The shunted blood never comes in contact with acinar units, whether or not these are ventilated, and for this reason the P_{O_2} of the arterial blood cannot be raised to a normal value (approximately 600 mm Hg) during inhalation of 100 per cent oxygen. In fact, when the shunt handles 10 per cent or more of the cardiac output, the arterial P_{O_2} will not rise above 400 mm Hg when 100 per cent oxygen is inhaled. All other mechanisms which produce hypoxemia can be fully corrected by the inspiration of 100 per cent oxygen, which replaces nitrogen in even the poorest ventilated acini. In true shunt, no matter how large, the P_{CO_2} always is normal or low, since additional ventilation effects removal of more carbon dioxide from acini which are perfused and ventilated. The inability of this compensatory hyperventilation to significantly improve uptake of oxygen is apparent on study of the oxygen- and carbon dioxide-dissociation curves (*see* Figure 1–41). Double the ventilation results in a decrease in P_{CO_2} from 40 to 20 mm Hg, with elimination of considerable amounts of carbon dioxide, whereas the increase in P_{O_2} that results from increase in ventilation produces an almost insignificant increase in arterial-blood oxygen content and saturation.

In most cases the hypoxemia and cyanosis that accompany pulmonary disease are due to $\dot{V}_A/\dot{Q}$ inequality. Chronic bronchitis and emphysema are the clinical conditions most commonly associated with this physiologic disturbance. The capillary blood that flows by underventilated acinar units is not fully saturated and does not release a normal amount of carbon dioxide, since the gradient between the P_{CO_2} of blood and of the acinus is reduced. However, again because of the difference in the dissociation curves, hyperventilation of well-ventilated acini, with consequent reduction in P_{CO_2} in such areas, increases the blood-to-acinus gradient and effects greater elimination of carbon dioxide from these areas. Consequently, patients with $\dot{V}_A/\dot{Q}$ inequality may have low, normal, or increased P_{CO_2}. The P_{CO_2} increases as the disease advances and the work of breathing results in greater production of carbon dioxide by the muscles of respiration than can be eliminated by the fewer normally functioning acini; or, perhaps more correctly, the P_{CO_2} rises when the patient, exposed to the discomfort of excessive respiratory effort, settles subconsciously for a higher arterial-blood P_{CO_2}—which, incidentally, is a compensatory mechanism, since it increases the P_{CO_2} gradient between blood and acinus. Patients with diseases that give rise to $\dot{V}A/\dot{Q}$ inequality can correct their hypoxemia and cyanosis by breathing 100 per cent oxygen, as oxygen replaces nitrogen in even the poorest ventilated areas. When carbon dioxide retention also is present, prolonged inhalation of oxygen increases the concentration of carbon dioxide in arterial blood, and confusion and coma may result. This further retention of carbon dioxide during oxygen breathing is due to removal of the carotid body's hypoxemic stimulus to ventilation.

Hypoxemia and carbon dioxide retention associated with hypoventilation is, in fact, only a gross example of $\dot{V}A/\dot{Q}$ abnormality. In diseases of the respiratory center itself and in neuromuscular disease affecting the thoracic cage, the overall decrease in ventilation may be generalized, resulting in underventilation despite normal perfusion, *i.e.*, the $\dot{V}A/\dot{Q}$ ratio may be reduced in every acinus in both lungs. When obesity is associated with hypoventilation, with resultant polycythemia, hypoxemia, and carbon dioxide retention, the $\dot{V}A/\dot{Q}$ inequality may be localized to the lung bases.[111] This form of hypoxemia may be readily corrected by the patient's taking a few deep breaths of even room air; this finding, together with good function-test values of bronchial flow, differentiates this condition from obstructive lung disease. The inhalation of 100 per cent oxygen by patients with general hypoventilation causes them to respond with further decrease in ventilation and its consequences, as occurs in other diseases which cause $\dot{V}A/\dot{Q}$ inequality.

Together with the analysis of arterial blood to determine oxygen saturation (or PO_2)—which indicates the abnormal physiologic process and, when combined with clinical information, aids in diagnosis—determination of the H^+ concentration (pH) of the blood is of the utmost importance. When carbon dioxide retention is present, the H^+ concentration indicates whether this represents acute respiratory failure or whether it is due to chronic failure in which the kidneys have had time and possess the ability to compensate by increasing bicarbonate. When the H^+ concentration is reduced and the PCO_2 also is below the accepted range, acute respiratory alkalosis is present. A normal concentration of H^+ with a decreased PCO_2 indicates chronic hyperventilation and a lapse of time sufficient for the development of compensation by the kidneys.

In addition to the respiratory causes of variation in PCO_2, H^+ concentration, and bicarbonate, some nonrespiratory (metabolic) processes produce acidosis and alkalosis and require secondary or compensatory under- or overventilation to return the acid-base balance to normal. A respiratory and nonrespiratory condition may act simultaneously; this occurs most commonly in cases of concurrent respiratory and cardiac arrest, when carbon dioxide accumulates and tissue hypoxia leads to an increase in formation of lactic acid.

Another somewhat confusing variation in acid-base balance is due to sudden improvement in ventilation in patients with chronic carbon dioxide retention. These subjects usually have emphysema and are in respiratory failure, their carbon dioxide retention being compensated by a secondary increase in bicarbonate. Artificial ventilation with a respirator produces a sudden fall in PCO_2, and, since the kidneys cannot adjust immediately, nonrespiratory alkalosis ensues. The same effect may be seen in cases of hypoventilation syndrome when arterial blood is drawn for gas analysis: the procedure induces sudden increase in ventilation, leading to a fall in PCO_2 but little change in the elevated level of bicarbonate.

Various changes in acid-base balance seen in our pulmonary function laboratory over a period of six months are illustrated by the short case histories depicted in Table 1–3.

SUMMARY. The amount of oxygen carried by the arterial blood can be measured by determining its content per 100 ml blood and dividing this by the total amount of oxygen the same blood can carry when exposed to oxygen (oxygen capacity): this ratio is known as the arterial oxygen saturation. A more reliable method is to measure the PO_2 of arterial blood with an electrode.

Most of the carbon dioxide is carried in the plasma as bicarbonate. The red blood cell, however, contains carbonic anhydrase, an enzyme which converts carbon dioxide into carbonic acid, H ions, and bicarbonate, the last of which crosses the cell membrane in exchange for chloride ions. Blood which contains reduced hemoglobin can carry more carbon dioxide, a circumstance which is ideal for assimilating carbon dioxide in the tissues and releasing it in the lungs.

Table 1–3. Disturbances in Acid-Base Balance

DIAGNOSIS \ TESTS AND NORMAL VALUES	*Age*	*Sex*	H^+	pH	P_{CO_2}	HCO_3^-	P_{O_2}	O_2Hb	CLINICAL HISTORY
			35 to 45 $M\mu$ Eq/L	7.35 to 7.45	35 to 45 mm Hg	22 to 28 mM/l	80 to 100 mm Hg	95 to 100 %	
Chronic Bronchitis and Emphysema	74	M	83	7.08	79	16.5		44	The patient was cyanotic and comatose when the first blood was drawn. A severe combined respiratory and nonrespiratory acidosis was found. Over the next 48 hours bicarbonate therapy slowly corrected the acidosis and oxygen the hypoxemia but the patient remained comatose with raised P_{CO_2} (bloods 2 and 3). An endotracheal tube was inserted and artificial ventilation was given by respirator. The fourth blood was taken 24 hours later while breathing room air. The P_{CO_2} was reduced considerably and the patient was left in mild nonrespiratory alkalosis.
			69	7.16	90	28		100	
			48	7.32	85	38		96	
			32	7.49	57	40		82	
Status Asthmaticus	45	F	36	7.44	51	32		83	The first and second blood were drawn at 48 hour intervals in a patient with an unusually prolonged attack of asthma. A compensated respiratory acidosis was found (both P_{CO_2} and bicarbonate raised). With intensive bronchodilator therapy the bronchospasm largely cleared and the patient was left with a mild nonrespiratory alkalosis. All bloods were taken while breathing room air.
			42	7.38	60	32		68	
			30	7.52	44	33.5	70	92	
Middle Cerebral Artery Thrombosis	58	F	31	7.51	29.2	22		90	The first blood was drawn following a sudden onset of coma and hemiplegia. The patient had aspirated. Respiratory alkalosis with mild hypoxemia was shown. The second blood was taken just before death with the patient breathing O_2. Hyperventilation persisted but a nonrespiratory acidosis had caused a fall in bicarbonate and the H^+ concentration was just above normal limits.
			46	7.34	16	9		100	
Liver Cirrhosis Terminal Renal Failure	62	M	50	7.30	29	14			This patient who was in a terminal state and died two days later showed a nonrespiratory acidosis (bicarbonate down and H^+ concentration up) partially compensated by hyperventilation (P_{CO_2} down).
Nephrolithiasis and Pyonephrosis Bronchopneumonia	72	M	53	7.28	38.5	16.8		92	A blood urea nitrogen of 205 mg per 100 ml indicated that this nonrespiratory acidosis (bicarbonate down, H^+ concentration up) was due to renal failure. Autopsy showed in addition bilateral bronchopneumonia which may account for his failure to produce a compensatory hyperventilation (P_{CO_2} unchanged).
Kidney Transplant	40	F	41	7.39	30	17.5			Since this blood was taken in a patient who had a recent kidney transplant and who showed slight nitrogen retention, it presumably represents a mild nonrespiratory acidosis with secondary hyperventilation. This picture is also quite compatible with a primary respiratory alkalosis with secondary renal compensation.
Pyloric Peptic Ulcer with Obstruction. Schizophrenia	49	F	30	7.52	59	43			This schizophrenic patient was admitted with persistent vomiting. A nonrespiratory alkalosis (bicarbonate up, H^+ concentration down) partially compensated by hypoventilation (P_{CO_2} up) was found. The vomiting was corrected and the acid-base balance was returned to normal (bloods not shown). Ten days later she was readmitted in a similar state and the attempt to compensate for the nonrespiratory alkalosis was reflected both in the lowered P_{O_2} and the raised P_{CO_2} (second blood). A pyloric ulcer was found and a subtotal gastrectomy was done. The final blood taken a few days after the operation showed a return of acid-base values to normal.
			26	7.58	60	54	61	87	
			38	7.42	34.5	21			

In diffuse infiltrative disease of the alveolar septa, arterial hypoxemia is due partly to $\dot{V}_A/\dot{Q}$ inequality and partly to diffusion defect and may be manifest only during exercise. Since carbon dioxide diffuses 20 times as readily as oxygen, in these diseases the diffusion defect is for oxygen only, and the P_{CO_2} is normal or low.

A true or absolute shunt results in hypoxemia without carbon dioxide retention. Patients with this condition hyperventilate and maintain low or normal levels of carbon dioxide. In chronic bronchitis and emphysema, hypoxemia is due mainly to $\dot{V}_A/\dot{Q}$ abnormality; the P_{CO_2} is low, normal, or high depending upon the patient's ability to hyperventilate and the presence of sufficient remaining functioning lung to compensate. Disease of the neuromuscular system or the respiratory center causes general hypoventilation and, therefore, hypoxemia and carbon dioxide retention. In the hypoventilation associated with obesity the $\dot{V}_A/\dot{Q}$ ratio at the lung bases appears to be grossly decreased; the unsaturation and carbon dioxide retention are readily corrected by the patients' taking a few deep breaths of even room air.

Measurement of the H^+ concentration of the arterial blood is an essential part of blood-gas analysis. Acute carbon dioxide retention is manifested by a rise in P_{CO_2} and a normal level of bicarbonate and, therefore, increase in H^+ concentration. Chronic carbon dioxide retention is accompanied by raised bicarbonate and normal H^+ concentration. Similarly, a low P_{CO_2} with decreased H^+ indicates acute hyperventilation and, with normal H^+ concentration, chronic hyperventilation. Secondary hyperventilation and hypoventilation may be initiated by nonrespiratory acidosis or alkalosis. Respiratory and nonrespiratory acid-base disturbances may occur simultaneously and can be interpreted only in full knowledge of the clinical situation.

DEVELOPMENT OF THE LUNG

The lung develops as a ventral outpouching of the foregut at 24 days of embryonic life. Intrauterine development is conveniently, if somewhat arbitrarily, divided into three periods: glandular, canalicular, and alveolar. The first, or *glandular phase*, lasts until the sixteenth week; during this time the primitive lung bud divides and redivides dichotomously and grows into the surrounding mesenchyme. At the end of this period bronchial divisions are nearly complete, but cartilage and bronchial glands continue to develop until the twenty-fourth week. The *canalicular period* is characterized by growth of the peripheral portion of the bronchial tree, producing the areas destined to become the acinus; during this period, capillaries grow into the lung, separating the epithelial cells into groups. The *alveolar phase* begins at about 24 weeks and is characterized by the development of evaginations of the terminal epithelium-lined tubes to form alveoli. At about 28 weeks, continuation of alveolar growth, attenuation of the lining epithelium, and capillary ingrowth produce an adequate area for gas exchange. Alveoli continue to develop through the remaining period of intrauterine life, until, at birth, there are approximately 24 million alveoli. For a long time it has been known that the lungs continue to grow after birth, but it is only recently that this has been determined quantitatively.[148] Alveoli continue to increase in number until the age of 8 years, when the full adult complement is reached. The alveolar surface area increases from 2.8 sq m at the time of birth to 32 sq m at age 8 years and continues to increase until the subject is 18 to 20 years of age. Alveolar surface area is linearly related to body surface area. The site and mode of alveolar development between birth and maturity are not known for certain. The adult complement of conducting airways is present at birth, and the alveolated structures (alveolar ducts and sacs) increase from 2 million at birth to 14 million at age 8 years (and maturity). This increase may be brought about by new growth of alveolar ducts and sacs, or by conversion of previously nonalveolated bronchioles to alveolar ducts and sacs, or a combination of the two.

THE NERVOUS SYSTEM

Sensory fibers from the lung run in the vagus and are derived from various sources. The bronchial epithelium contains nerve endings which are sensitive to tactile stimulation and which continue as far as respiratory bronchioles. Stretch receptors are present in the lamina propria, muscle, and cartilage of the bronchi. The pulmonary veins are particularly well supplied, and the terminals of the subendothelial nerves probably are chemoreceptors. Branches associated with venules lie in septa in the periphery of lobules, and it is likely that these are sensitive to stretch. Pressor receptors are present in the muscle of pulmonary arteries and veins.

The motor supply is derived from both sympathetic and parasympathetic systems. The sympathetic supply is from the second, third, and fourth thoracic sympathetic ganglia, and the parasympathetic, through the vagus, forms peribronchial and perivenous ganglia. Motor supply in the bronchial tree extends as far as the terminal bronchioles, and in the pulmonary artery and vein to the limit of muscle. The bronchial arteries also have a rich nerve supply.

THE PLEURA

Morphology

The lung is encased by the visceral pleura, a stable membrane which is separated from the limiting membrane of the lung by a layer of loose connective tissue. The pleura is only loosely attached to the limiting membrane—the two are readily separated in the plane of the subpleural connective tissue, and fluid or air may collect in this layer. Expansion of the lung is restricted to some extent by the limiting membrane and the pleura, as evidenced by the close correlation between total lung volume at full inspiration during life and lung volume after death, even with high transpulmonary pressures. Further, impressions caused by the heart and great vessels remain after death, despite inflation to high transpulmonary pressure.

The pleura consists of a thin superficial layer or endopleura and a denser, deeper layer known as the chief layer. The superficial layer consists of a delicate sheet of elastic and collagenous fibers, in no particular pattern, underlying a sheet of mesothelial cells. These cells are thin and flattened, a few microns thick and about 30μ in diameter; they may swell to become cuboidal and can multiply rapidly. The chief layer of the pleura, which is responsible for its mechanical stability, consists of dense collagenous and elastic tissue. The chief layer crosses intralobar fissures with the superficial layer.

The subpleural connective tissue consists of loose connective tissue which is a continuation of the pulmonary interstitial tissue. Lymphatic channels, veins, arteries, and a rich capillary network are present in this layer, which is also referred to as the vascular layer of the pleura. Irregularly placed bands of collagenous and elastic fibers extend perpendicularly or obliquely from the chief layer to the limiting membrane, although, as mentioned previously, these two layers are but loosely bound together.

Roentgenology

The combined thickness of the parietal and visceral pleural layers over the convexity of the lungs and over the diaphragmatic and mediastinal surfaces is insufficient to render these layers roentgenographically visible in the normal human subject. The diaphragmatic and mediastinal pleura, even if uniformly thickened to a moderate degree, is never visible, since its water density precludes roentgenographic separation from the contiguous diaphragm and mediastinum. Over the convexity of the lungs, however, thickening of only slight degree (1 to 2 mm, for example) can be appreciated because of the greater density of contiguous ribs. Such an appearance is evidence of either current pleural disease or residual thickening from past disease.

In the interlobar regions, contiguous layers of visceral pleura are roentgenographically visible because of the presence of air-containing lung on both sides. Interlobar fissures become visible when the x-ray beam passes tangentially along their surfaces; when visualized, these constitute a valuable aid to the assessment of disease of the pulmonary lobes which form them. Much of our knowledge of the incidence of roentgenographic visualization of normal and accessory fissures was supplied by Felson,[69, 119] whose review of the chest roentgenograms of large numbers of normal human subjects provided accurate statistics on this and other aspects of normal roentgen anatomy.

Fissures

Normal Interlobar Fissures. Fissures form the contact surfaces between

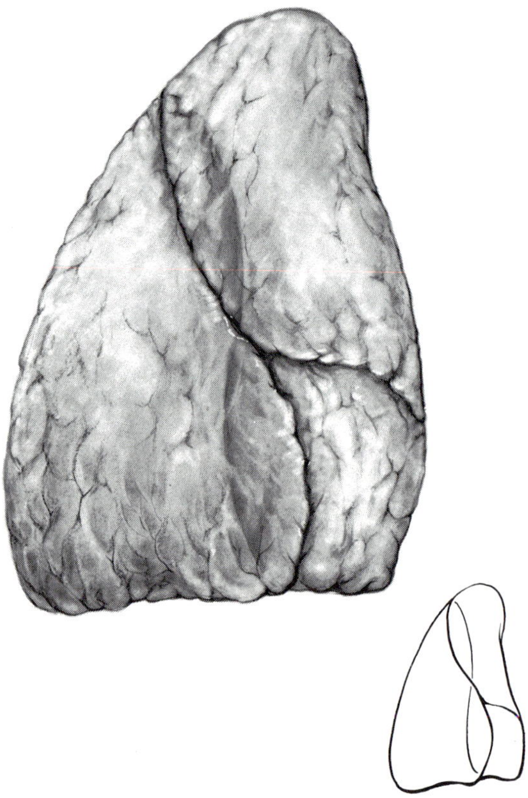

Figure 1–42. **Interlobar Fissures, Right Lung.** A drawing of the right lung from its lateral aspect reveals the major fissure to be shaped like an airplane propeller, its upper half facing forward and slightly laterally and its lower half forward and slightly medially.

pulmonary lobes. They vary greatly in depth from complete separation of lobes to no more than a superficial slit not more than 1 to 2 cm deep in the surface of the lung. The depth of interlobar fissures is important: The less complete a fissure line the larger the bridge of lung parenchyma connecting two contiguous lobes; such parenchymal bridges provide a ready pathway for collateral air-drift or for the spread of disease from one lobe to another, thereby creating roentgenographic signs that may give rise to erroneous conclusions. Therefore, in assessing certain diseases, due consideration should be given the depth of interlobar fissures.

Interlobar surfaces seldom appear flat when viewed anatomically. For example, major fissures face forward and slightly outward in their upper half, whereas in their lower half they face forward and slightly medially (similar to an airplane propeller) (Figure 1–42). Similarly, the minor fissure, although in a generally horizontal plane, may make a double curve, the medial portion being convex upward and the lateral half convex downward, thus creating a shallow S configuration. These curvatures explain the relative infrequency with which fissures are visualized along their entire length; however, should complete roentgenographic visualization be desired, it is necessary only to rotate the patient slightly into different obliquities to bring all portions of the fissures into profile. In some cases the configuration of the entire fissure can be extrapolated or interpolated quite accurately from the appearance of short segments.

THE OBLIQUE (MAJOR) FISSURE. This fissure (Figure 1–43), which separates the upper and middle lobe from the lower lobe, begins at or about the level of the fifth thoracic vertebral body and extends obliquely downward and forward, roughly paralleling the sixth rib, ending at the diaphragm a few centimeters behind the anterior pleural gutter. The major fissures are incomplete at the mediastinal surface of the lungs much more frequently than is generally realized; Schall and Hoffman are said by Shanks and Kerley[120] to have found failure of the main fissure to reach the mediastinal surface above or below the hilum in 50 per cent of lungs. In lateral roentgenographic projection, if portions of both major fissures are visualized, the laterality of each can be determined from the junction of the right fissure with the horizontal fissure or by the relationship of both to the hemidiaphragms (the left hemidiaphragm being identifiable by its relationship to the gastric air bubble).

THE HORIZONTAL (MINOR) FISSURE. This fissure (Figure 1–43), which separates the anterior segment of the right upper lobe from the right middle lobe, lies in a roughly horizontal plane at about the level of the fourth rib anteriorly. As has been indicated, its contour is variable—to a point, in fact, at which Felson concluded on the basis of a study of 1000 normal subjects that significance cannot be attached to displacement of the fissure unless it is of major degree.[69] Anatomically the minor fissure rarely reaches the mediastinum, and then only in its anterior portion; despite this, one of the more constant relationships of the minor fissure noted by Felson roentgenograph-

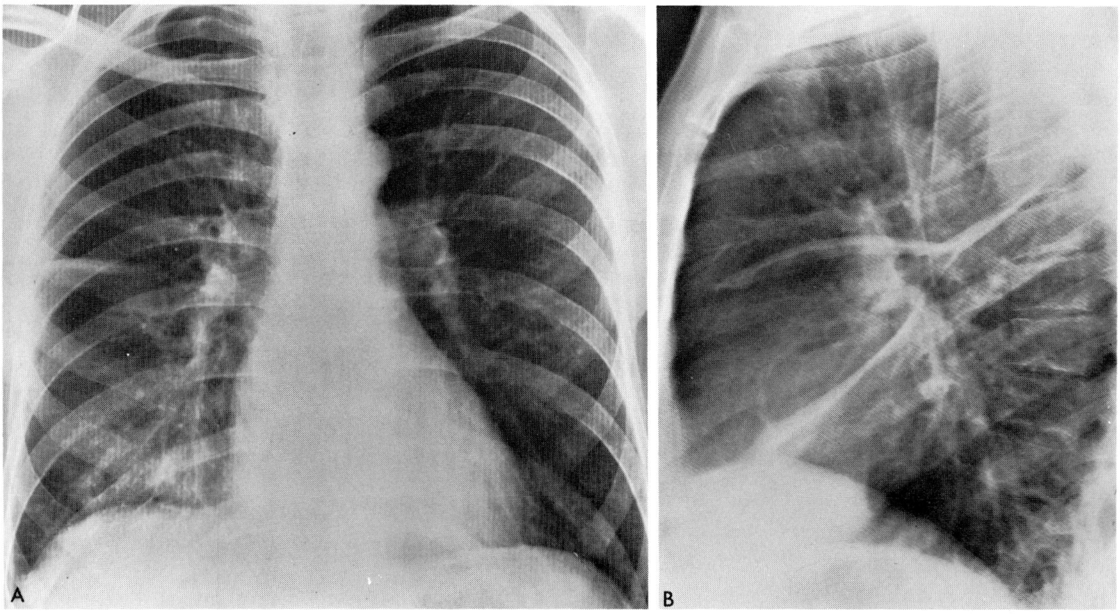

Figure 1–43. **Interlobar Fissures, Right Lung.** The presence of minimal interlobar effusion renders the fissures clearly visible in posteroanterior (*A*) and lateral (*B*) roentgenograms.

ically was its medial termination at the lateral margin of the inferior pulmonary artery, about 1 cm distal to the origin of the artery. Reports of the roentgenographic visualization of the minor fissure in normal subjects vary considerably: Felson[69] saw it in 56 per cent, Ritter and Eyband[121] in 70 per cent, and Simon[122] in over 80 per cent.

ACCESSORY (SUPERNUMERARY) FISSURES. It is important to realize that any segment of lung may be partially or completely separated from its adjacent segments by an accessory pleural fissure. The incidence anatomically is much higher than is generally appreciated, amounting to about 50 per cent of lungs, according to von Hayek.[15] These fissures vary in their degree of development from superficial slits in the lung surface not more than 1 to 2 cm deep to complete fissures which extend all the way to the hilum. More often than not these accessory fissures are of little more than academic interest roentgenologically; when well developed, however, their recognition is important for two reasons: (1) the segment they subtend may be the only site of disease whose spread is prevented by the presence of a fissure and (2) when a fissure is present in a specific anatomic location, such as between the superior and basal segments of the right lower lobe, it may be mistaken for the minor fissure between upper and middle lobes and thus create confusion in interpretation.

Perhaps the best known of the accessory fissures, although of no known pathologic significance, is the *azygos fissure* (the mesoazygos), which is created by downward invagination of the azygos vein through the apical portion of the right upper lobe (Figures 1–44 and 1–45). The familiar curvilinear shadow which extends obliquely across the upper portion of the right lung is formed by four pleural layers (two parietal and two visceral), since the azygos vein is anatomically external to the parietal pleura and thus invaginates four layers in its downward course. The fissure terminates in the "tear-drop" shadow caused by the vein itself at a variable distance above the right hilum. Felson states that this fissure is visible in 0.4 per cent of chest roentgenograms.[119]

According to Boyden,[181] the bronchial supply of the azygos lobe is somewhat variable: either the apical (B^1a) or the anterior (B^1b) subsegmental branch of the apical bronchus is always present; in larger lobes, both these subsegments or the apical subsegments of the apical (B^1a) and posterior (B^3a) segmental bronchi may be present. The importance of the anomaly roentgenologically (in addition to the reasons previously stated) lies in the fact that the apical pleural surfaces fail to separate in the presence of pneumothorax.

A fissure line, traditionally referred to as "the inferior accessory fissure of the right lower lobe," is present rather frequently anatomically; von Hayek[15] found it in 30 per cent of lungs, and Schaffner is said to have seen it in 45 per cent of 210 lungs studied at necropsy.[123] This accessory fissure is of variable depth, from a superficial slit to a complete fissure extending all the way to the hilum; when complete, it isolates the medial basal segment of the lower lobe which thus becomes the inferior accessory or retrocardiac lobe. Roentgenographically, a fissure line extending superiorly and slightly medially from the inner third of the right hemidiaphragm is visible in approximately one-third of subjects, according to Felson,[119] but whether this line represents the anatomic inferior accessory fissure is open to some question. Although Felson feels that they are the same, Simon[124] regards the roentgenographic shadow as the medial reflection of the normal chief fissure between the middle and lower lobes visualized in profile. We have no personal evidence to support either contention, but on the strength of the evidence presented, we are inclined to favor the latter interpretation.

Another accessory fissure with which the roentgenologist should be familiar is that which separates the superior segment from

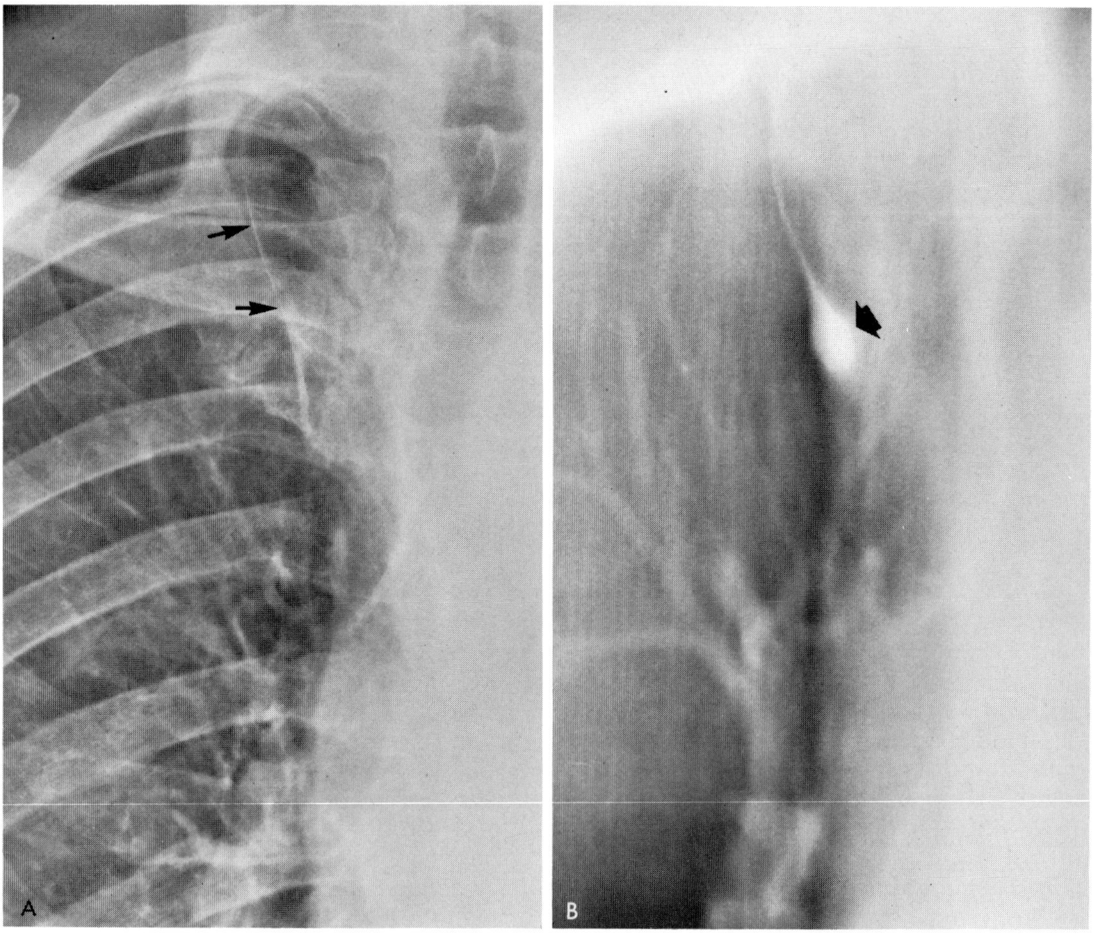

Figure 1–44. **Accessory Fissure of the Azygos Vein.** On a standard roentgenogram in posteroanterior projection (*A*), the fissure can be identified as a curvilinear shadow (arrows) extending obliquely across the upper portion of the right lung, its lower end some distance above the right hilum. A tomographic section with the patient in the supine position (*B*) permits better visualization of the tear-drop shadow of the vein (arrow) because of distension.

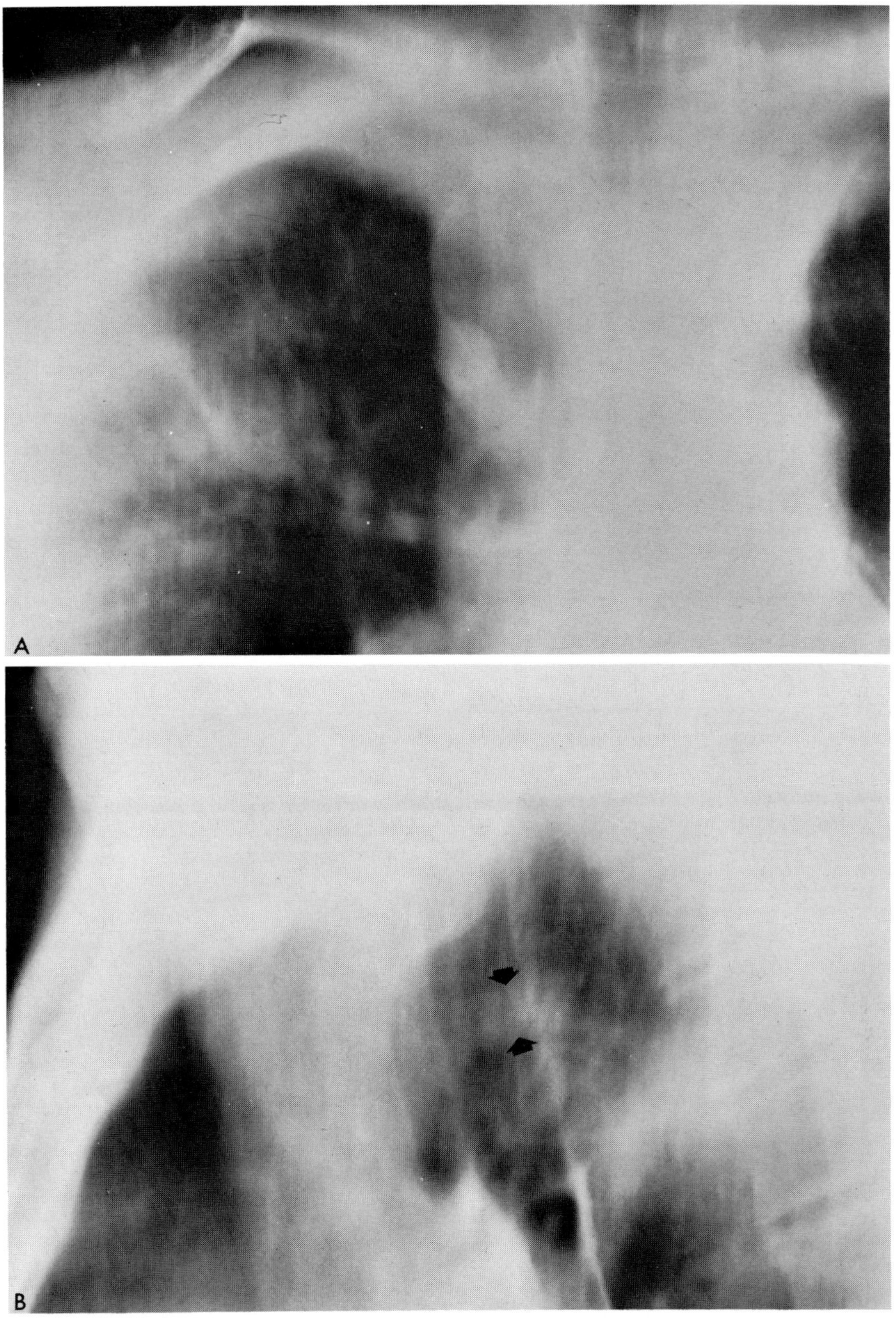

Figure 1–45. **Accessory Fissure of the Azygos Vein (in Congestive Heart Failure).** *A*, A tomographic section of the upper thorax in anteroposterior projection, supine position, reveals a slightly distended azygos vein at the lower end of a thickened fissure. The patient was in cardiac decompensation. *B*, In lateral projection, the shadow of the vein (arrows) can be seen lying in a horizontal plane extending anteriorly to the shadow of the brachiocephalic vessels.

the basal segments of the lower lobes, more commonly on the right (Figure 1–46). Since this fissure commonly lies in a horizontal plane at the same level as the minor fissure, the two may be confused in a frontal roentgenogram, although their separate anatomic positions may be clearly established on lateral or oblique roentgenography. Boyden[125] states that another accessory fissure, which separates the lingula from the remainder of the left upper lobe, occurs in 8 per cent of cases; when this is present the arrangement of fissures is a mirror image on the two sides.

In recent years a line shadow has been described which lies in a vertical plane in the lower portion of the chest of some infants and children; this is termed the "vertical fissure line."[126-128] The line is visible on frontal projections of the thorax and extends from the lateral portion of the diaphragmatic dome upward and slightly medially, roughly parallel to the thoracic wall, terminating at the level of the horizontal fissure. It has been identified in both lungs but more often in the right. Several theories have been postulated to explain this fissure line; most of the evidence indicates that it represents the lower portion of the major fissure which has been thrown into profile because of alteration in position of the middle and lower lobes. Precisely how or why this positional change occurs is not clear, but the major importance of the line lies in its recognition as such and in its differentiation from the visceral pleural line in pneumothorax. It seems likely that, ultimately, this will prove to be similar to the phenomenon seen in the chest roentgenograms of adults, when partial collapse of the lower lobe has caused downward and medial displacement of the major fissure, thus rendering it visible in profile in frontal projection.

Physiology

The visceral and parietal pleura form smooth membranes which facilitate the movement of the lungs within the pleural space. The membranes secrete and absorb pleural fluid which renders movement easy.

Pressures

Pressure within the pleural cavity represents the difference between the elastic forces of the chest wall and of the lungs. Lung tissue has a natural tendency to recoil and will continue to do so even after the lungs have been removed from the body. Thus, even at the end of a maximal expiration (residual volume) the lungs tend to collapse. By contrast, the chest wall rests at about 55 per cent of vital capacity; below this volume it has a natural tendency to expand, and above this it tends to recoil inward toward the resting position. At resting lung volume (at the end of a quiet expiration, or functional residual capacity) the chest wall is still below its resting position of 55 per cent of the vital capacity. Thus, the chest wall's tendency to expand

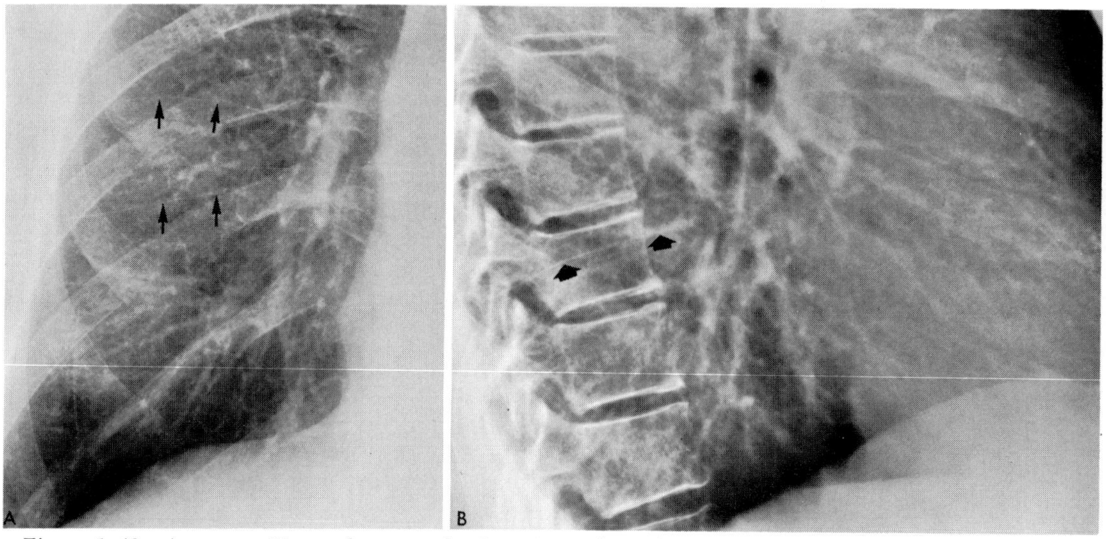

Figure 1–46. **Accessory Fissure between the Superior and Basal Segments of the Right Lower Lobe.** *A,* In a posteroanterior projection of the lower half of the right lung two horizontal fissures can be identified, the superior (upper arrows) representing the normal minor fissure and the inferior (lower arrows) representing an accessory fissure between the superior and basal bronchopulmonary segments of the right lower lobe. *B,* In lateral projection, only the accessory fissure is visualized (arrows).

outward is opposed by an equal and opposite force from the lungs. At this point pleural pressure is about −5 cm H_2O. However, pleural pressure is not uniform throughout the pleural cavity, although its precise variation and its cause and effects are not certain.[101] Pleural pressure is more negative at the apex of the pleural cavity than at the base, and the gradient probably is about 0.2 cm H_2O per centimeter vertical height—although a steeper pressure gradient has been suggested recently.[129] The gradient is not uniform and is greater over the upper than the lower zones of the lung. It is gravity-dependent, since it is reversed in subjects in the head-down position.

The effects of this gradient have been demonstrated by Milic-Emili and others,[101] who have shown that the upper lung zones are more expanded than the lower in subjects in the upright position at all lung volumes other than total lung capacity. The lower lung zones expand more than the upper during inspiration, and this is reflected by the greater ventilation of the lower zones in healthy, young, erect subjects. Regional volume behavior of the lung has been compared to that of an easily extensible coiled spring.[101] If the spring is held at its upper end so that it is acted upon only by the force of gravity, the coils will be further apart at the upper than at the lower end of the spring: this is analogous to the greater alveolar volume in upper than in lower lung zones. If the spring is lengthened by applying a weight at the bottom, the distances between coils will increase until they are equal: The change in distance between the coils is greater at the lower end, corresponding to the greater change in volume at the bottom of the lung.

Fluid Formation and Absorption

In normal man, transudation and absorption of fluid within the pleural cavity follow the Starling equation and depend upon a combination of hydrostatic pressures, colloid osmotic pressures, and tissue pressures. The latter are not known, but knowledge of the first two forces suggest that, in health, fluid is formed at the parietal pleura and absorbed at the visceral pleura (Figure 1–47). The net hydrostatic pressure which forces fluid out of the parietal pleura results from the hydrostatic pressure in the systemic capillaries that supply the parietal pleura (30 cm H_2O) and the pleural pressure (−5 cm H_2O at functional residual capacity). Thus, the net hydrostatic drive is 35 cm H_2O pressure. The colloid osmotic pressure in the systemic capillaries is 34 cm H_2O, and that of the pleura[130] approximately 8 cm H_2O, which yield a net drive of 26 cm colloid osmotic pressure from the pleural space to the capillaries of the parietal pleura. The balance of these forces (35 − 26 cm = 9 cm H_2O) is directed from the parietal pleura to the pleural cavity. The visceral pleura, other than over the mediastinal surfaces, is supplied by pulmonary artery capillaries, whose hydrostatic pressure is approximately 11 cm H_2O. Other pressures remain roughly constant. Thus, the net hydrostatic pressure from visceral pleura toward pleural cavity is 16 cm H_2O (11 cm less −5). The osmotic colloid pressures remain constant, with a pressure of 26 cm away from the pleural cavity. The net effect of these forces is a drive of 10 cm H_2O (26 − 16 cm) toward the visceral pleural capillaries. The preceding is an oversimplification since it ignores tissue pressures, the permeability of the mesothelial

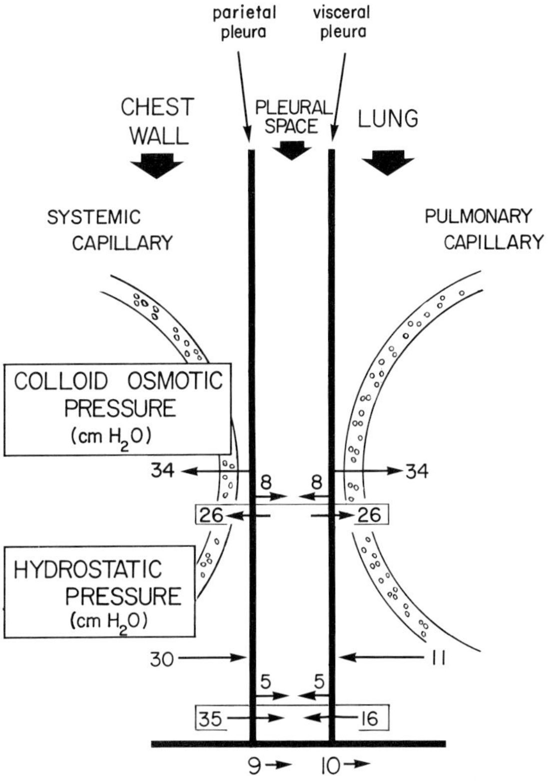

Figure 1–47. **Diagrammatic Representation of the Pressures Involved in the Formation and Absorption of Pleural Fluid.** *See* text for description.

layer, and pressures within the lymphatics through which excess fluid will be absorbed. However, this estimate of the forces that act on pleural fluid is supported by the findings of Agostoni and associates[131] that the visceral pleura of the dog absorbs saline at a pressure related to these forces.

It should be appreciated that, in health, pleural fluid is of low protein content, amounting to approximately 100 mg per 100 ml;[176, 177] such a low concentration permits formation of fluid by the parietal pleural capillaries and its absorption by the visceral pleural capillaries according to Starling's principles. When protein concentration rises sufficiently, to a figure in excess of approximately 1.0 g per 100 ml, the effect of colloid osmotic pressure of the visceral pleural capillaries is reduced to negligible proportions, and the only route of absorption of pleural fluid will be via the lymphatics by bulk flow.[178, 180] Since parietal pleural lymphatic vessels pass through the diaphragm and intercostal muscles, it might be thought that movement of the chest wall might increase lymphatic flow and speed of absorption from the pleural space; Burgen and Stewart[180] have shown that such occur in unanesthetized dogs. Stewart[176] has found that the rate of absorption of protein-high fluid in humans falls significantly during the night; he has postulated that a decrease in rate and depth of respiration during sleep might account for this phenomenon.

It is apparent that abnormal amounts of fluid may accumulate when there is an increase in hydrostatic pressure, a decrease in colloid osmotic pressure, or an increase in capillary permeability. Increased hydrostatic pressure causes the pleural effusion that occurs in heart failure; increased capillary permeability is responsible in inflammatory and neoplastic disease of the pleura. The *site* of accumulation of fluid is dependent upon hydrostatic forces and, to some extent, upon capillary attraction between the lung and the thoracic wall.

THE LYMPHATIC SYSTEM

Lymphatics of the Lungs and Pleura

Although the entire cardiac output passes through the lungs and the lung has a rich lymphatic supply, lymphatic flow from the lungs is small compared with that which drains the systemic circulation. The pleural lymphatics are of variable size and number and occur much more frequently over the lower than the upper lobes (Figure 1–48*A*). Lymph flows in them for a variable distance on the surface of the lung and then passes centrally to the hilum, via the septal, perivenous, and peribronchial lymphatics. Alveoli and alveolar sacs have no lymphatic ducts, which start in the region of the alveolar ducts and respiratory bronchioles and flow centripetally in the bronchovascular sheath toward the hilum (Figure 1–48*B*). Lymphatic channels also drain the periphery of the lung lobules, where they run in the lobular septa along with the pulmonary veins (the site of Kerley "B" lines). The lymph flow in these also is toward the hilum, except in the subpleural region, where pleural lymphatics occasionally dip into the lung and then return to the surface to become pleural again.[175] Anastomotic channels exist between the perivenous lymphatics and those in the bronchovascular sheath; they measure up to 4 cm in length and usually lie approximately midway between the hilum and the periphery of the lung (it is distention of these communicating lymphatics that results in Kerley "A" lines). Numerous valves, 1 to 2 mm apart, direct the flow of lymph in both pleural and intrapulmonary lymphatics.

Normal lymph nodes may be found in the substance of the lung, far from the hilum: Trapnell[112] found intrapulmonary lymph nodes in five of 28 lungs in which he could outline the deep lymphatic channels. Occasionally, a peripheral lymph node may present as a coin lesion.[113]

Lymphatics of the Mediastinum

Although our major concern is with lymphatic drainage of the lungs and pleura, involvement of the mediastinal lymph nodes occurs not infrequently in diseases arising in the breast, the chest wall, the diaphragm, or intra-abdominal or retroperitoneal structures; therefore, a thorough understanding of all afferent and efferent drainage pathways and of nodal anatomy is imperative. Individual patterns of lymph node enlargement may supply an important clue to the origin or nature of a disease process arising inside or outside the thorax.

Intrathoracic lymph nodes usually are divided into two main anatomic groups, the parietal and visceral mediastinal nodes. The former drain the thoracic wall and certain extrathoracic tissues, and the latter are concerned almost entirely with intrathoracic structures. For purposes of roentgenographic description, however, such a classification is less useful than one based on subdivision of groups of nodes in relation to the three mediastinal compartments. Since extensive communications exist not only between the parietal and visceral groups of nodes but also within the visceral group itself, an anatomic description based on mediastinal zones possesses considerable merit.

The Anterior Mediastinal Compartment

Two chains of lymph nodes are present in the anterior compartment, the sternal and the anterior mediastinal (visceral) groups (Figure 1–49).

THE STERNAL (ANTERIOR PARIETAL OR INTERNAL MAMMARY) GROUP. This group is situated extrapleurally. The nodes are scattered along the internal mammary arteries and behind the anterior intercostal spaces and costal cartilages bilaterally. Two or three may be directly retrosternal. These nodes are variable in number but occur more consistently superiorly. Their afferent channels drain the upper anterior abdominal wall, the anterior thoracic wall, the anterior portion of the diaphragm, and the medial portions of the breast. They communicate with the visceral group of anterior mediastinal nodes and the cervical nodes, and their main efferent channels are the right lymphatic duct or bronchomediastinal duct on the right and the thoracic duct on the left.

THE ANTERIOR MEDIASTINAL (PREVASCULAR) GROUP. This group comprises

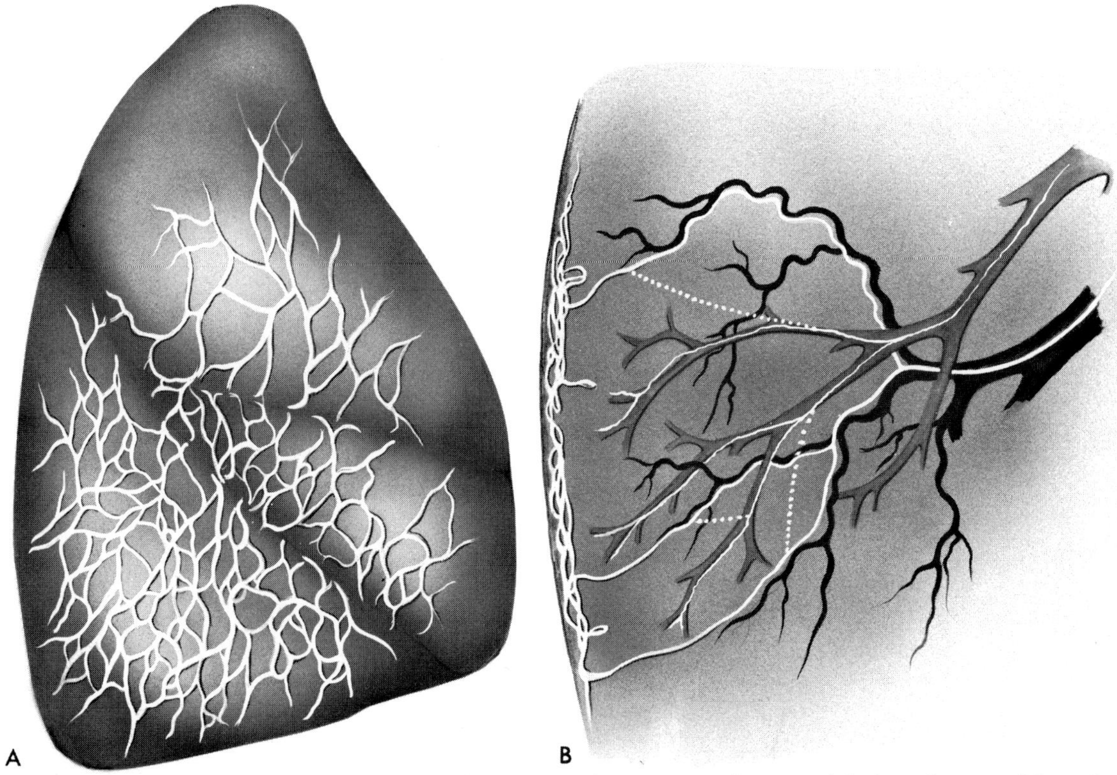

Figure 1–48. **The Lymphatic Drainage of the Pleura and Lungs.** *A,* A drawing of the lateral aspect of the right lung shows the pleural lymphatics to be much more numerous over the lower half of the lung than over the upper. *B,* In a coronal section through the midportion of the lung, lymphatic channels from the pleura enter the lung at the interlobular septa and extend medially to the hilum along venous radicals (dark shaded vessels); lymphatic channels originating in the peripheral parenchyma extend medially in the bronchovascular bundles (light shaded vessels). Communicating lymphatics (dotted lines) extend between the peribronchial and perivenous lymphatics.

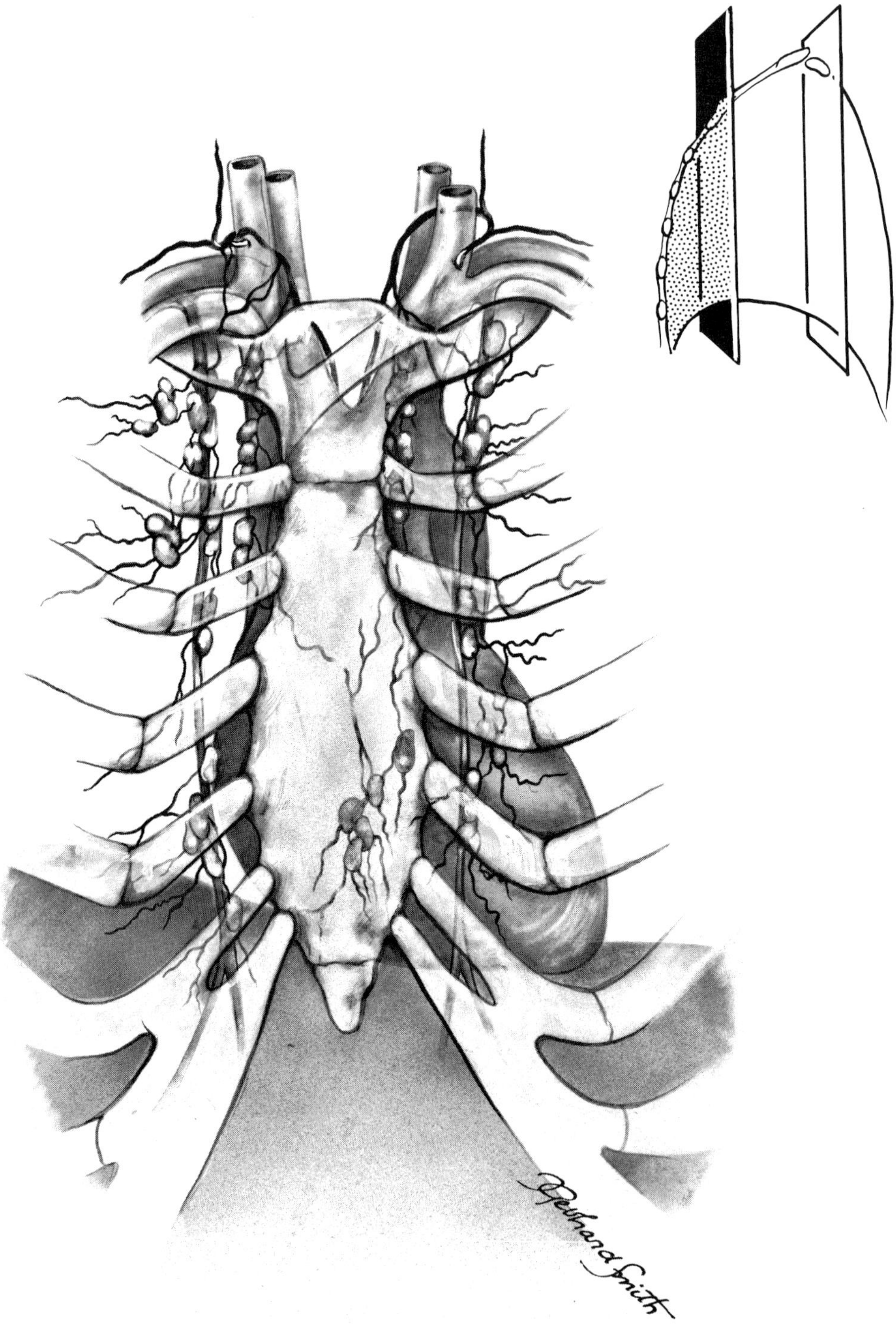

Figure 1–49. **Anterior Mediastinal Lymph Nodes.** The nodes illustrated are chiefly those of the anterior parietal group scattered along the internal mammary arteries and behind the anterior intercostal spaces and costal cartilages bilaterally. The prevascular (visceral) group relate to the superior vena cava and innominate vein on the right and to the aorta and carotid artery on the left.

the second group of nodes in the anterior mediastinal compartment; they belong to the visceral collection. A few nodes are situated posterior to the sternum in the lower thorax, but the majority are grouped in the prevascular areas bilaterally, along the superior vena cava and innominate vein on the right and in front of the aorta and carotid artery on the left side. A few lie anterior to the thymus behind the manubrium. These nodes drain most of the structures situated in the anterior mediastinum, including the pericardium, part of the heart, the thymus, the thyroid, the diaphragmatic and mediastinal pleura, and the anterior portions of the hila bilaterally. Their efferent channels drain via the bronchomediastinal trunk or thoracic duct.

The Posterior Mediastinal Compartment

Groups of nodes belonging to both the parietal and the visceral chains lie in the posterior mediastinum (Figure 1–50).

THE INTERCOSTAL (POSTERIOR PARIETAL) GROUP. This group lies laterally, in the intercostal spaces, and medially, in the paravertebral areas adjacent to the heads of the ribs. Both groups drain the intercostal spaces, the parietal pleura, and the vertebral column. They communicate with the posterior mediastinal group of visceral nodes and possess efferent channels which drain to the thoracic duct from the upper portions of the thorax and to the cisterna chyli from the lower thoracic area.

THE POSTERIOR MEDIASTINAL GROUP. This group of visceral nodes is situated along the lower esophagus and descending aorta. They possess afferent channels from the posterior portion of the diaphragm, the pericardium, the esophagus, and directly from the lower lobes of the lungs. They communicate with the bifurcation group of tracheobronchial nodes and drain mainly via the thoracic duct.

The Middle Mediastinal Compartment

This compartment also includes parietal and visceral components.

THE PARIETAL GROUP. This group is of little importance roentgenologically. The nodes are situated mainly around the pericardial attachment to the diaphragm and drain the diaphragm itself and portions of the liver. Efferent pathways pass anteriorly to the sternal or anterior mediastinal nodes and posteriorly to the posterior mediastinal nodes.

From the roentgenologic point of view the other lymph nodes in the middle mediastinal compartment undoubtedly constitute the most important group in the thorax: the *tracheobronchial, carinal,* and *bronchopulmonary* nodes (Figure 1–51). Although these groups freely communicate with one another, in many cases involvement is predominantly in one group.

THE TRACHEOBRONCHIAL NODES. These nodes are scattered along the lateral aspects of the trachea and in the tracheobronchial angles and are more numerous on the right than on the left. One node which is fairly constant in position is situated in the right tracheobronchial angle contiguous to the azygos vein; this is commonly referred to as the azygos node. Afferent channels arise from the bronchopulmonary and bifurcation nodes, from the trachea and esophagus, and from the right or left lung directly without diversion via the bronchopulmonary or bifurcation nodes. Direct communication exists with the anterior and posterior groups of visceral mediastinal nodes. The efferent channels are the bronchomediastinal trunk on the right and the thoracic duct on the left.

THE BIFURCATION (CARINAL) NODES. These nodes are situated along the anterior and inferior aspects of the carina and extend downward along the medial aspects of the main bronchi to the origin of the lower-lobe bronchi bilaterally. They receive afferent drainage from the bronchopulmonary nodes, the anterior and posterior mediastinal nodes, the heart, pericardium, and esophagus, and directly from both lungs. Efferent drainage is to the right tracheobronchial group.

THE BRONCHOPULMONARY NODES. These nodes are numerous bilaterally but variable in number. They lie in the angles between the bronchial bifurcations in the hilar regions and are closely related to the arteries and veins. Their afferent supply is from all pulmonary lobes, and efferent drainage is to the bifurcation and tracheobronchial nodes.

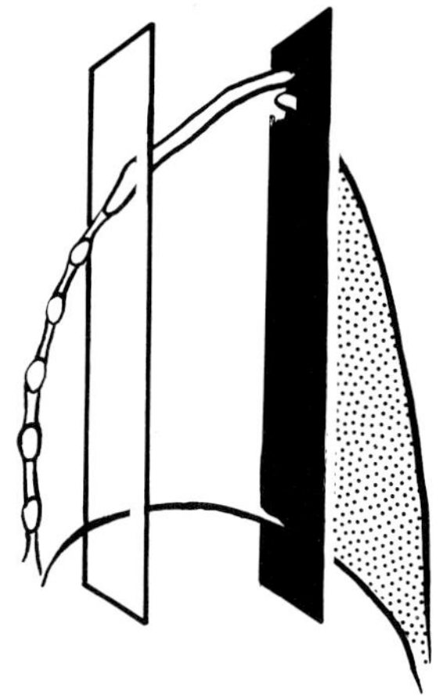

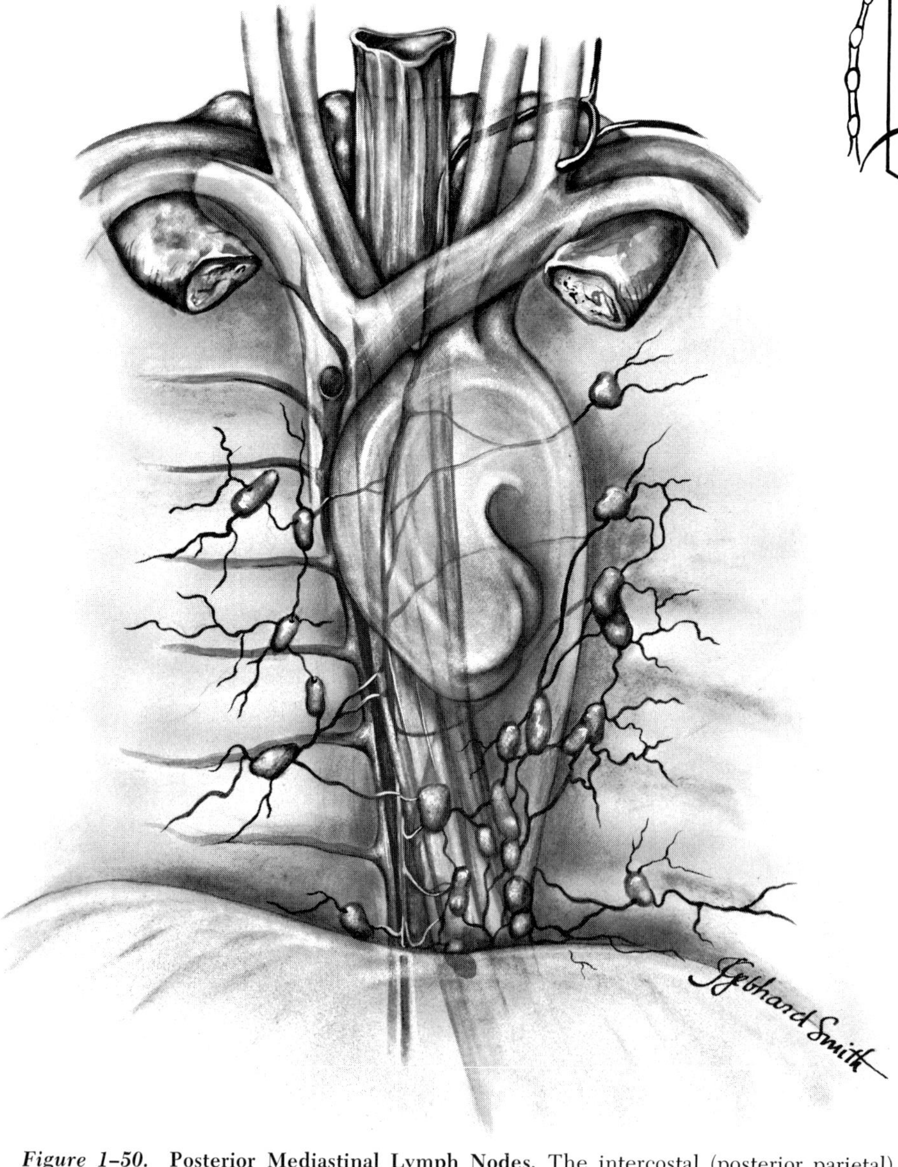

Figure 1–50. **Posterior Mediastinal Lymph Nodes.** The intercostal (posterior parietal) group lies laterally, in the intercostal spaces, and medially, in the paravertebral areas adjacent to the heads of the ribs. The visceral group of posterior mediastinal nodes is situated along the lower esophagus and descending aorta.

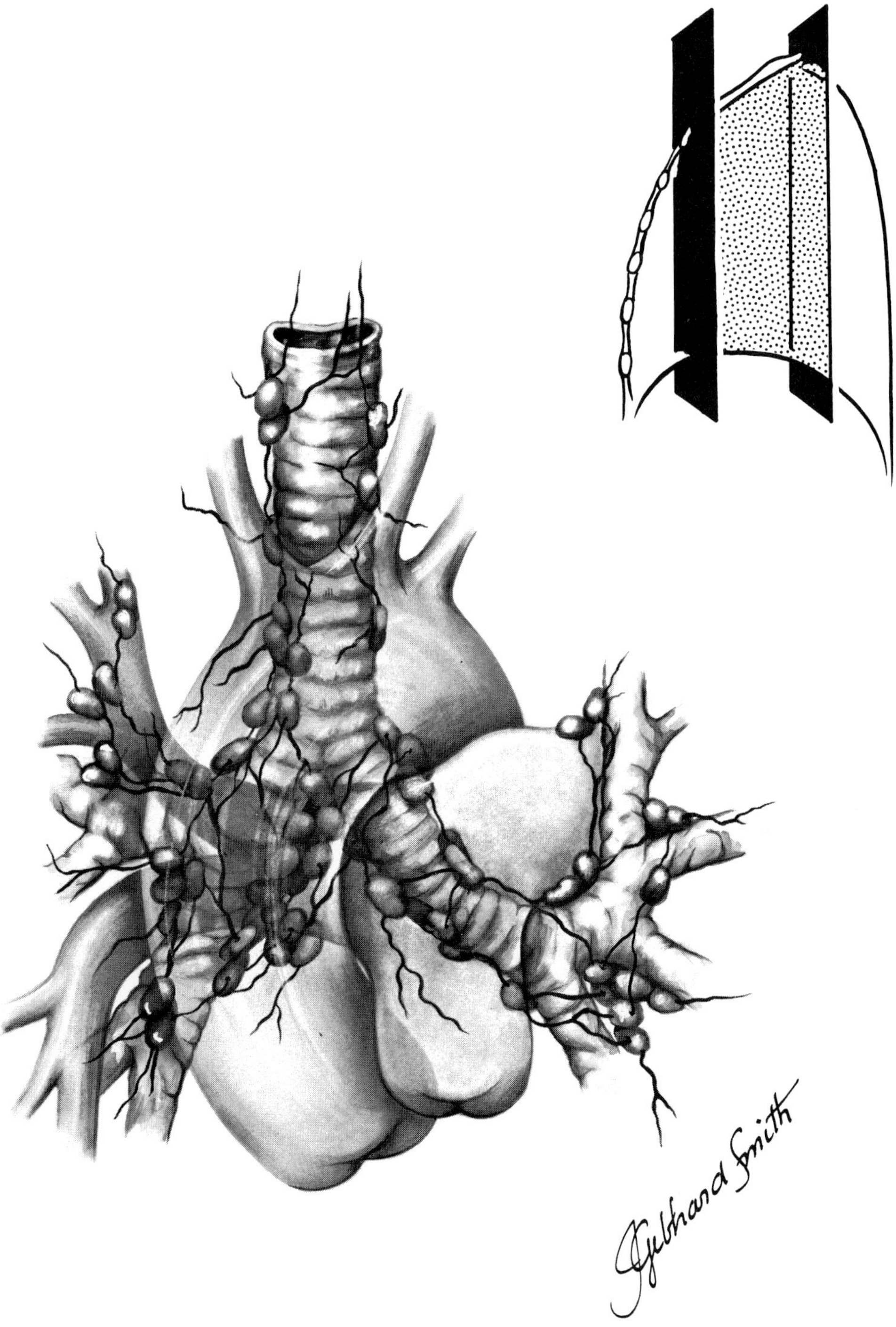

Figure 1–51. **The Middle Mediastinal Lymph Nodes.** Only the visceral group of nodes are depicted, consisting of the tracheobronchial, carinal and bronchopulmonary nodes. *See* text for description.

Patterns of Lymphatic Drainage of the Lungs

The location of enlarged lymph nodes within the mediastinum may be of importance in determining the site of origin within the lungs of an infectious or neoplastic process. Much of our knowledge of patterns of regional lymph node drainage from the lung derives from Rouvière's treatise[114] on the anatomy of the human lymphatic system, published in 1938, which was based on necropsy studies of 200 fetuses, neonates, and children. Many of his observations were subsequently confirmed by McCort and Robbins[115] and by Nohl.[116] Rouviere subdivided the lungs into three main drainage areas, the superior, middle, and inferior, without correspondence to pulmonary lobes.

On the Right Side

On the right side, in the superior area, lymph drains directly into the paratracheal and upper bronchopulmonary nodes. The middle zone drains directly into the paratracheal nodes, the bifurcation nodes, and the central group of bronchopulmonary nodes. The inferior zone drains into the inferior bronchopulmonary and bifurcation nodes and the posterior mediastinal chain. Thus, on the right side, all the lymph drains eventually via the right lymphatic duct.

On the Left Side

On the left side, Rouvière[114] stated that, in the superior area, lymph drains into both the prevascular group of anterior mediastinal nodes and directly into the left paratracheal nodes. The middle zone drains mainly via the bifurcation and central group of bronchopulmonary nodes and partly directly into the left paratracheal group. The inferior zone drains into the bifurcation and inferior bronchopulmonary nodes and into the posterior mediastinal chain. Thus, according to Rouvière,[114] the superior portion and part of the middle zone drain via the left paratracheal nodes into the thoracic duct, and lymph drainage from the remainder of the left lung empties eventually into the right lymphatic duct.

The "crossover" phenomenon was long thought to be of diagnostic and therapeutic importance in diseases which originated in the middle or lower portion of the left lung. However, recent investigations have cast some doubt on the validity of the phenomenon in adult patients. For example, in a study of 1000 consecutive necropsies, Klingenberg[117] found 17 cases of primary carcinoma of the left lung, only one of which had heterolateral prescalene-node metastases; unfortunately, the sites of origin in the left lung were not stated. Similarly, Baird[118] performed bilateral prescalene-node biopsies in 218 patients of whom 110 had bronchogenic carcinoma; the direction of lymphatic spread within the mediastinum was cephalad and usually ipsilateral, irrespective of the location of the primary growth. Contralateral spread occurred uncommonly and with about equal frequency from the two lungs.

On the strength of these observations, it is reasonable to conclude that prescalene-node biopsies should always be performed first on the same side as the pulmonary disease; should this prove negative, contralateral biopsy may *occasionally* be productive.

THE MEDIASTINUM

The mediastinum constitutes a compartmented septum or partition which divides the thorax vertically (Figures 1–52 and 1–53). For descriptive purposes, it is traditionally divided into two major compartments, the superior and the inferior, the latter being subdivided into anterior, middle, and posterior compartments. Since each compartment contains anatomic structures which are almost unique to it, many of the affections to which the mediastinum is subject tend to occur *predominantly* in one or other compartment; thus, this anatomic subdivision has considerable merit. However, of the four compartments, the superior possesses little practical importance as a separate division; defined as that area bounded superiorly by the thoracic inlet and inferiorly by a line drawn from the angle of Louis (the manubriosternal angle) to the intervertebral disc between the fourth and fifth thoracic vertebrae, it not only contains structures which extend across this imaginary line into the inferior mediastinum but also some which extend into it from below. In this book, therefore, the entire mediastinum from the thoracic inlet to the diaphragm is considered to possess three major compartments, the an-

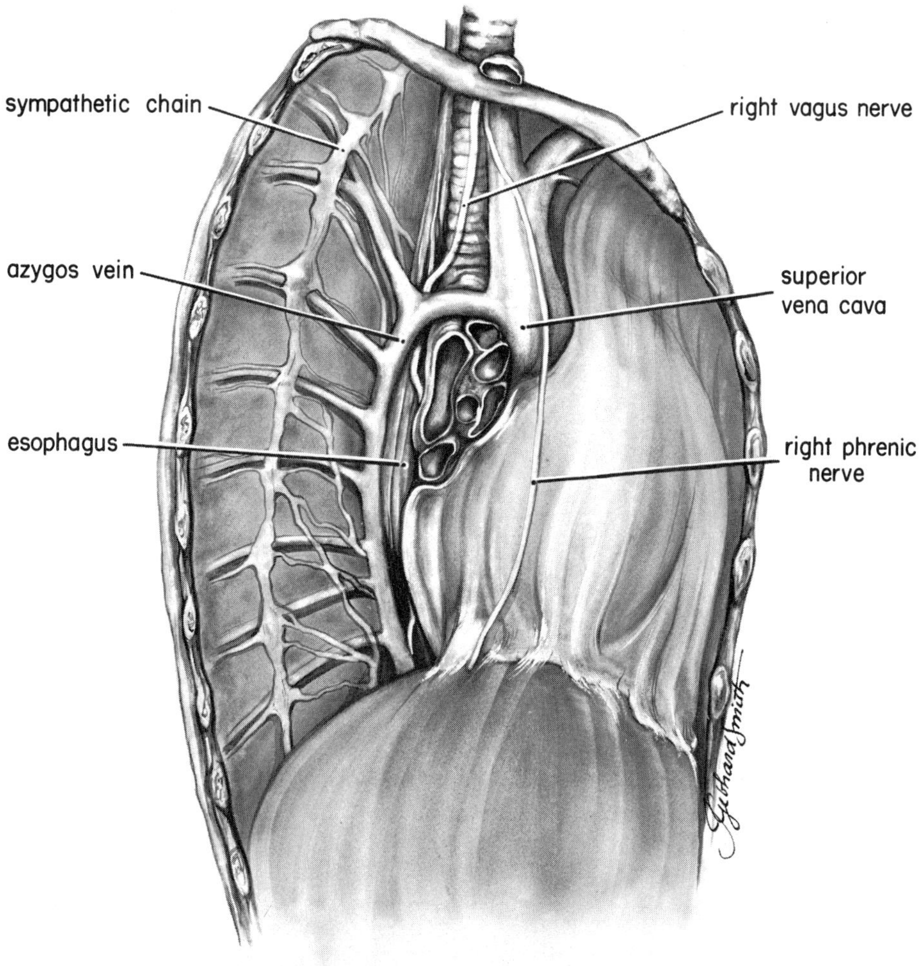

Figure 1–52. **The Mediastinum – Right Lateral Aspect.** In the anterior mediastinum, the thymus gland is not depicted. In the middle mediastinal compartment can be identified the pericardium overlying the heart, the superior vena cava, the phrenic nerve, the upper half of the vagus nerve, a cross section of the bronchi and vessels in the hilum, and the horizontal portion of the azygos vein. In the posterior compartment are depicted the esophagus and the azygos vein with its intercostal tributaries. The sympathetic chain lies along the lateral aspect of the vertebral column (and therefore not truly mediastinal).

terior, middle, and posterior, without reference to a separate superior compartment.

The anatomic boundaries of the mediastinum are as follows: *lateral*, the parietal pleural reflections along the medial aspects of both lungs; *superior*, the thoracic inlet; *inferior*, the diaphragm; *anterior*, the sternum; and *posterior*, the anterior surfaces of the thoracic vertebral bodies.

The Mediastinal Compartments

The Anterior Mediastinal Compartment

The anterior mediastinal compartment (Figures 1–52 and 1–53) is bounded anteriorly by the sternum and posteriorly by the pericardium, aorta, and brachiocephalic vessels. It contains the thymus gland and the anterior mediastinal lymph nodes, including both parietal and visceral groups. It is relatively narrow, particularly inferiorly, where the pericardium overlying the right ventricle is in contact with the lower portion of the sternum.

The Middle Mediastinal Compartment

The middle mediastinal compartment (Figures 1–52 and 1–53) contains the pericardium and heart, the ascending and transverse arch of the aorta, the superior and

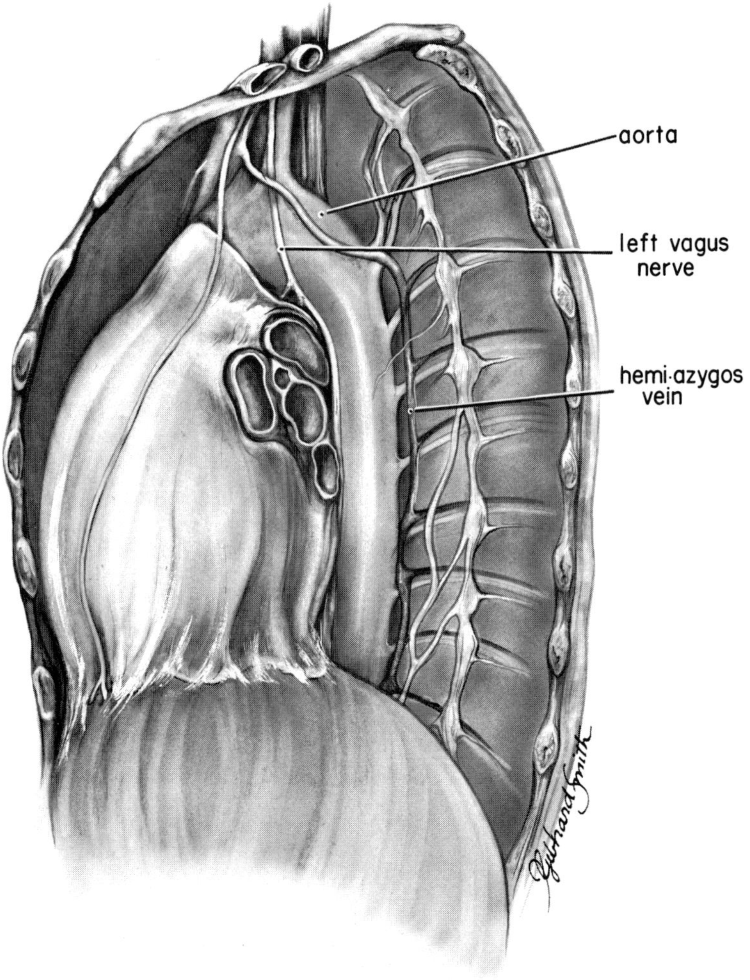

Figure 1–53. **The Mediastinum—Left Lateral Aspect.** No anatomic structures are depicted in the anterior mediastinum. In the middle mediastinal compartment, in addition to the structures already described in Figure 1–52, are the ascending and transverse arch of the aorta and the brachiocephalic arteries. Most of the vagus nerve can be identified. In the posterior mediastinal compartment, the descending thoracic aorta and hemiazygos veins can be seen.

inferior vena cavae, the brachiocephalic arteries and veins, the phrenic nerves and upper portion of the vagus nerves, the trachea and main bronchi and their contiguous lymph nodes, and the pulmonary arteries and veins.

The Posterior Mediastinal Compartment

The posterior mediastinal compartment (Figures 1–52 and 1–53) lies between the pericardium and the anterior aspect of the vertebral column. It contains the descending thoracic aorta, the esophagus, the thoracic duct, the azygos and hemiazygos veins, the sympathetic chains and the lower portion of the vagus nerves, and the posterior group of mediastinal lymph nodes. Since the posterior limit of the mediastinum is formed by the anterior surface of the vertebral column, the paravertebral zones and posterior gutters are not included in the mediastinum.

It is important to recognize certain lines which are visible within the mediastinal contour on well-exposed frontal roentgenograms of the chest, since deviations in their pattern may supply important clues to the presence of disease. The reflection of the pleura from the posterior thoracic wall onto the *right* side of the mediastinum is smooth and uninterrupted by protruding structures except for the right atrium, the superior vena cava above, and the inferior vena cava below. It is invisible, therefore, on frontal roentgenograms of the chest. By contrast, on the left side, the descending thoracic aorta protrudes slightly laterally in the posterior mediastinal compartment, causing lateral displacement of the mediastinal pleura posterior to it. This creates *the paraspinal line* (Figure 1–54), a shadow first described by Brailsford,[132] consisting of a longitudinal density projected about midway between the outer border of the descending thoracic aorta and the vertebral column, extending from the aortic arch above to the diaphragm below.[133] In cases of right-sided aorta, when the descending aorta passes downward on the right, the paraspinal line appears on the right side. As might be expected, elongation of the thoracic aorta displaces the paraspinal line laterally; similarly, deformity of the line may be an important indication of disease of various structures in the posterior mediastinum and vertebral column.

Three other contour lines are visible sometimes on frontal roentgenograms of the chest, particularly when high kilovoltage or tomographic techniques are employed. *The anterior mediastinal line*[134] is a thin linear density measuring no more than 1 to 2 mm in diameter, projected over the air column of the trachea for a distance of a few centimeters distal to the plane of the junction of the manubrium and the body of the sternum (Figure 1–55). This line, which represents the anterior mediastinal septum, is produced by the combined shadows of the visceral and parietal pleura of the two contiguous upper lobes, possibly with a small amount of areolar tissue interposed between. It may be confused with a somewhat similar density, the *posterior mediastinal line* (Figure 1–56*A*), which is slightly higher and is formed by apposition of the pleural surfaces of the two lungs in the supra-aortic triangle of the posterior mediastinal compartment.[135] This linear density also projects over the air column of the trachea and usually is situated at a higher level than the anterior mediastinal line, its center being in the plane of the upper surface of the manubrium. Its right side generally is slightly concave. Since the esophagus descends through the supra-aortic triangle, it is probable that this organ

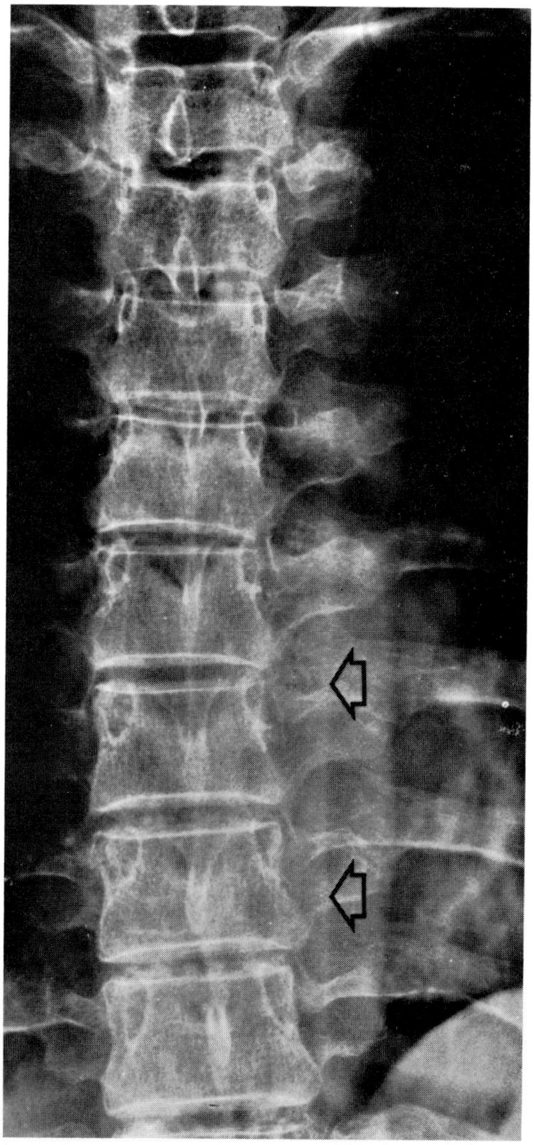

Figure 1–54. **The Paraspinal Line.** A roentgenogram of the mediastinum in anteroposterior projection, supine position; normal 42-year-old male. A longitudinal shadow (arrows) extending from the arch of the aorta to the diaphragm is projected about midway between the lateral border of the descending aorta and the vertebral column; this shadow is caused by the paravertebral mediastinal pleura being displaced laterally by the descending aorta.

contributes to the formation of the posterior mediastinal line (Figure 1–56*B* and *C*)—a concept emphasized by Cimmino, who designated the line the "esophageal-pleural stripe";[136-138] he saw it in 25 of 200 consecutive chest roentgenograms.

The lower lobes may come into close apposition in the inferior portion of the pos-

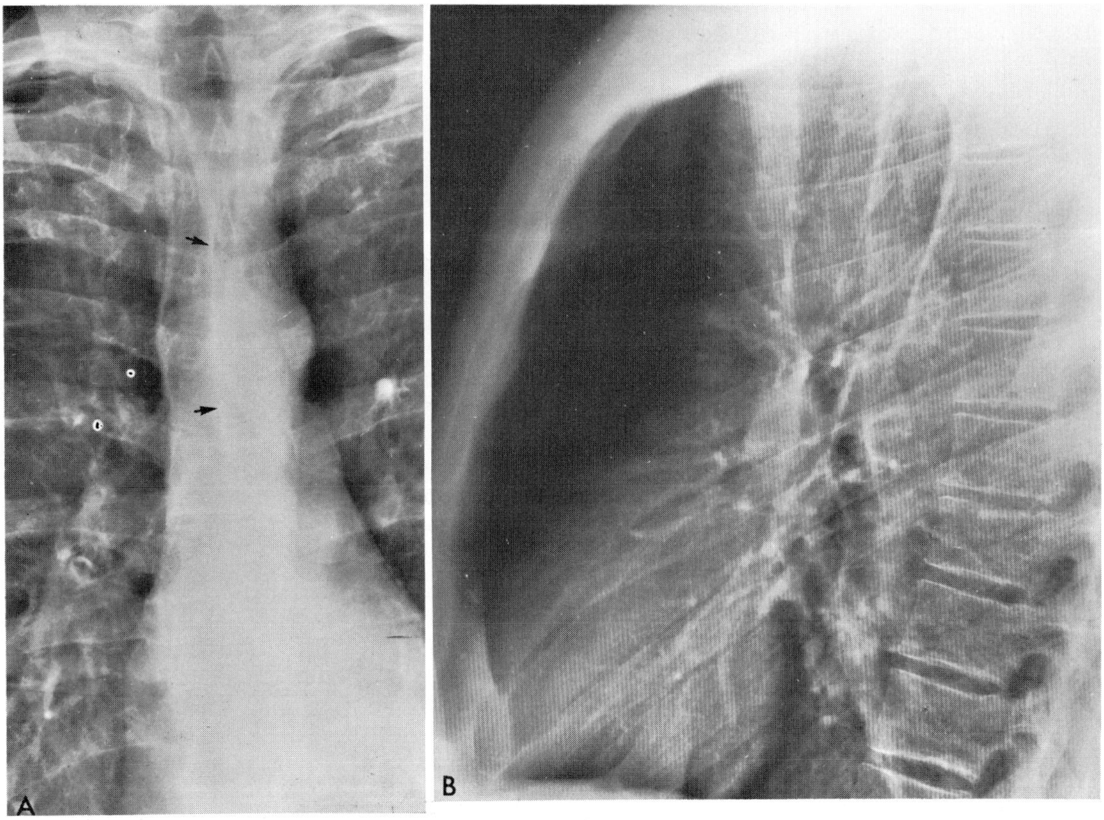

Figure 1–55. **The Anterior Mediastinal Line.** *A*, A roentgenogram of the chest in posteroanterior projection reveals a thin line shadow projected over the air column of the trachea (arrows). It is caused by the combined shadows of the visceral and parietal pleura in the anterior mediastinal septum. *B*, In the lateral projection, note the deep retrosternal air space.

terior mediastinal compartment, in a triangular area of the mediastinum posterior to the heart and anterior to the spine, which is known as the retrocardiac space or the space of Holzknecht. In this region, the mediastinum deviates slightly to the left of midline; the esophagus, lying in the central portion of this mediastinal septum, is related intimately to the adjacent pleural surface covering the right lower lobe, thus creating what Cimmino refers to as the *inferior esophageal-pleural stripe*[137, 138] (Figure 1–56A). In normal subjects this measures 3 to 5 mm in width with the esophagus distended;[138] greater widths than this may indicate the presence of esophageal disease.

Detailed definition of the anterior mediastinal line and the superior and inferior esophageal-pleural stripes has been obtained by Lodin[139] through the use of axial transverse tomography.

The Heart

It is clearly beyond the scope of this book to discuss the heart in any detail. However, it is important to recognize that certain deviations in the normal roentgen anatomy of the cardiovascular silhouette may give rise to confusion.

Position

In a frontal roentgenogram of the normal chest (*see* Figure 1–67, page 92), the position of the heart in relation to the midline of the thorax depends greatly upon the build of the patient. As has been pointed out by Simon,[122] the heart shadow of an asthenic patient is almost exactly midline in position, projecting only slightly more to the left than to the right of the midline. In those of more sthenic build, the heart lies more to the left than to the right (in the range of three-quarters to one-quarter).

These statements assume, of course, that the roentgenograms are exposed with the lungs fully inflated.

Size and Contour

Due chiefly to the influence of systole and diastole, both size and contour may vary in any one patient from one examination to another, even when all examinations are made with an identical degree of lung inflation. In a series of 200 normal subjects studied by Simon,[122] the maximal difference in transverse cardiac diameter on successive examinations was 2 cm (in one patient only), and the average variation was 0.5 cm for the whole group.

When the influence of systole and diastole is controlled (which may be accomplished easily by exposures of one second or longer), the major influences on cardiac size and contour are three-fold. (1) *The height of the diaphragm*, which, in turn, is influenced by the degree of pulmonary inflation: obviously, the lower the position of the diaphragm, the longer and, therefore, narrower, the cardiovascular contour will become. (2) *Intrathoracic pressure*: this factor influences not only cardiac size but also the appearance of the pulmonary vascular pattern. (3) *Body position*: assuming equality of all other factors, the heart is broader when the subject is recumbent than when he is erect. The physiologic and

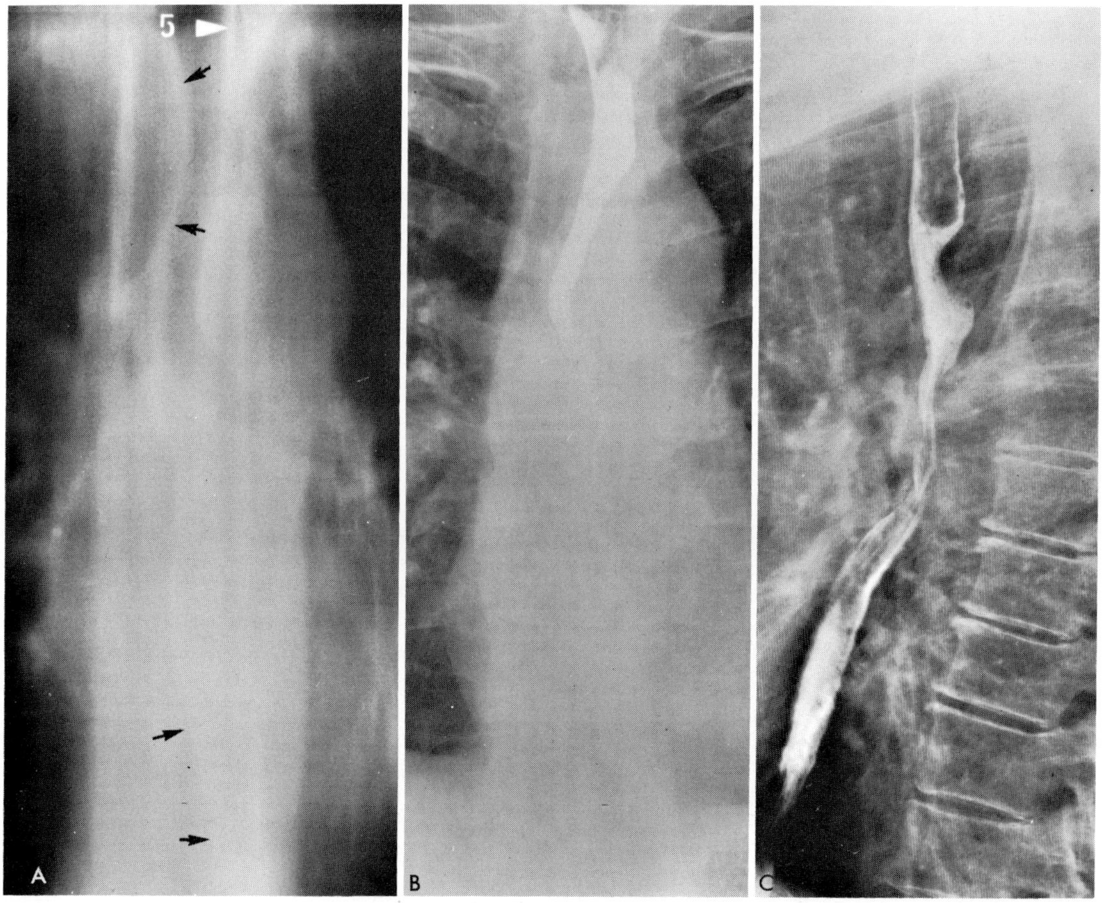

Figure 1–56. **The Posterior Mediastinal Line and the Superior and Inferior Esophageal–Pleural Stripes.** *A*, A tomographic section of the posterior mediastinum reveals a longitudinal curvilinear shadow (upper arrows) projected over the air column of the trachea; this line is formed by apposition of the pleural surfaces of the two lungs posteriorly in the supra-aortic triangle. It is probable that the esophagus contributes to the formation of this line as revealed in the posteroanterior and lateral roentgenograms of the chest (*B* and *C*) with barium in the esophagus–thus the designation superior esophageal–pleural stripe. The inferior esophageal–pleural stripe seen in *A* (lower arrows), is situated in the retrocardiac space of Holzknecht and is formed by the right mediastinal pleura; the esophagus is intimately related to this pleural surface.

roentgenographic effects of variation in intrathoracic pressure and body position are discussed in detail later in this book.

It is to be emphasized that standardization of all these influences is essential to accurate comparison of heart size on films taken at different times. Methods of standardization may vary but could well include the following criteria. The patient should be in the erect position in posteroanterior projection, at a standard 6-ft focus-film distance, with the lungs inflated to total lung capacity (or some other easily reproducible level of lung inflation, measured by spirometry), at a known intrathoracic pressure (preferably atmospheric pressure, which is attained by suspending respiration with glottis open and specifically without a Valsalva maneuver), and with a radiation exposure of one second or longer. It is clear that the time required to perform such an examination renders it impracticable for routine use: These parameters are outlined only to stress the importance of their control if comparisons of heart size on successive examinations are to be accurate.

Other Aspects of Mediastinal Configuration

Physiologic accumulations of fatty tissue commonly occur bilaterally in the cardiophrenic recesses, producing an obtuse angular configuration of the inferior mediastinum at its junction with the diaphragm (Figure 1–57). Usually their density is slightly less than that of the heart, allowing identification of cardiac borders through them. These pleuropericardial fat shadows should not be misinterpreted as cardiac enlargement or as mediastinal or diaphragmatic masses of possible importance.

In a posteroanterior roentgenogram of the chest (*see* Figure 1–67, page 92), the right mediastinal border from the right atrium to the lung apex is formed by the superior vena cava and the innominate vein. In the normal subject, providing the chest is correctly centered, the ascending aorta contributes nothing to the mediastinal contour. The extreme superomedial portion of the right hemithorax in the plane of the second and third posterior interspaces may be formed by the right subclavian artery. On the left side, the silhouette of the superior mediastinum above the arch of the aorta is formed mostly by the subclavian artery.[140]

The Azygos Vein

The azygos vein usually is visible in frontal chest roentgenograms of normal subjects as a slightly flattened elliptical shadow in the right tracheobronchial angle (Figure 1–58*A*). Fleischner and Udis[141] measured the vein from its outer border to the contiguous tracheal air column on teleroentgenograms of erect subjects and recorded a maximum normal transverse diameter of 6.0 mm. Evidence accumulated since this first report suggests that this figure may be a trifle low; for example, Felson[182] states that a transverse diameter of 10 mm may be normal, and we have personally observed several normal subjects whose vein measured 9 mm. Perhaps the definitive work on the subject, however, is the recent report of Keats and his associates[183] who measured the diameter of the arch of the azygos vein of 100 men and 100 nonpregnant women and recorded the following results: in men, minimum size 3 mm, maximum size 7 mm, average size 4.91 mm; in nonpregnant women, minimum size 3 mm, maximum size 7 mm, average size 4.87 mm. It seems reasonable to conclude that while normal subjects may occasionally have an azygos vein measuring up to 9 or 10 mm in diameter, the vast majority will be 7 mm or less; if a patient has a vein of more than 7 mm in diameter, one should exercise caution in labeling it as normal before excluding all causes of azygos enlargement.

Of considerable interest in this last report[183] was the wide range of measurements and increased average size of the azygos arch observed in 100 pregnant women: the minimum size was unchanged at 3 mm, but the maximum size was 15 mm and the average 7.14 mm. This normal effect of pregnancy should be borne in mind when considering the differential diagnosis of azygos vein enlargement.

Doyle and his associates,[142] who used a tomographic technique with a shorter focus-film distance and with the patient supine, (Figure 1–58*B*) measured the maximum diameter of the azygos vein in 48 normal subjects and plotted this against several parameters, including age, sex, weight, height, and body surface area. The only significant correlation was between body weight and azygos vein diameter. Standardization of all measurements to a body

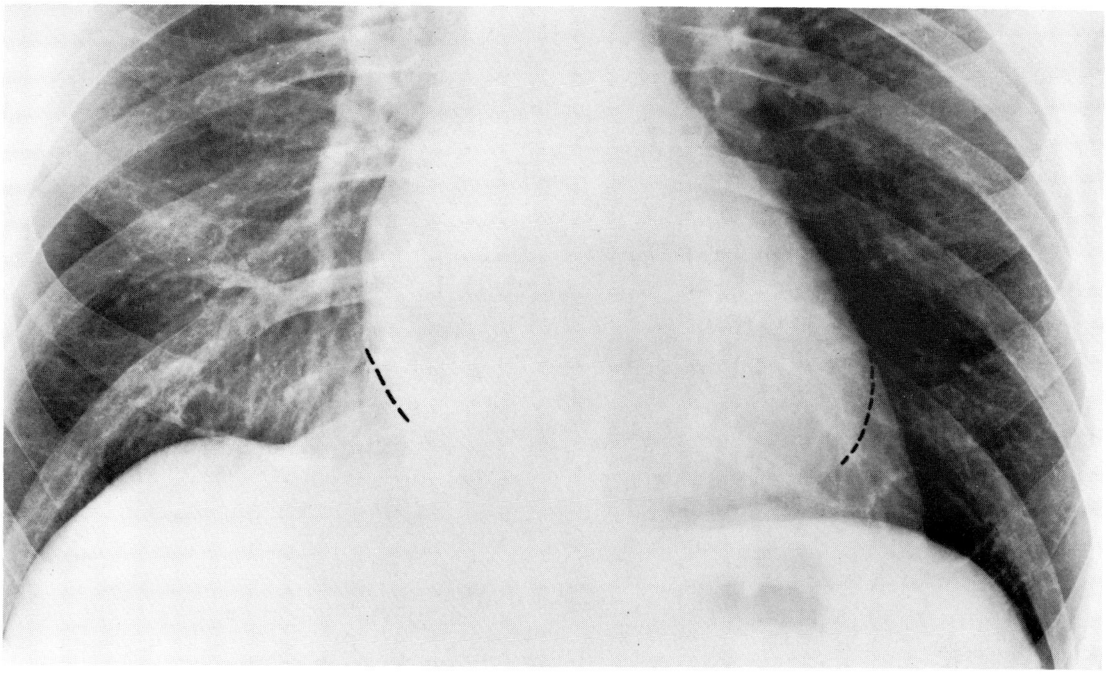

Figure 1–57. **Pleuropericardial Fat Shadows.** In this posteroanterior roentgenogram of the lower half of the thorax, physiologic accumulations of fatty tissue can be identified in the cardiophrenic recesses bilaterally. The borders of the heart are indicated by dotted lines.

Figure 1–58. **The Azygos Vein Shadow.** *A*, A roentgenogram in the erect position shows the azygos vein as an elliptical-shaped shadow projected in the right tracheobronchial angle (arrows). *B*, In the same subject, a tomographic section of the mid-mediastinum in the supine position demonstrates a much larger vein shadow (arrows) owing to distension brought about by the supine body position.

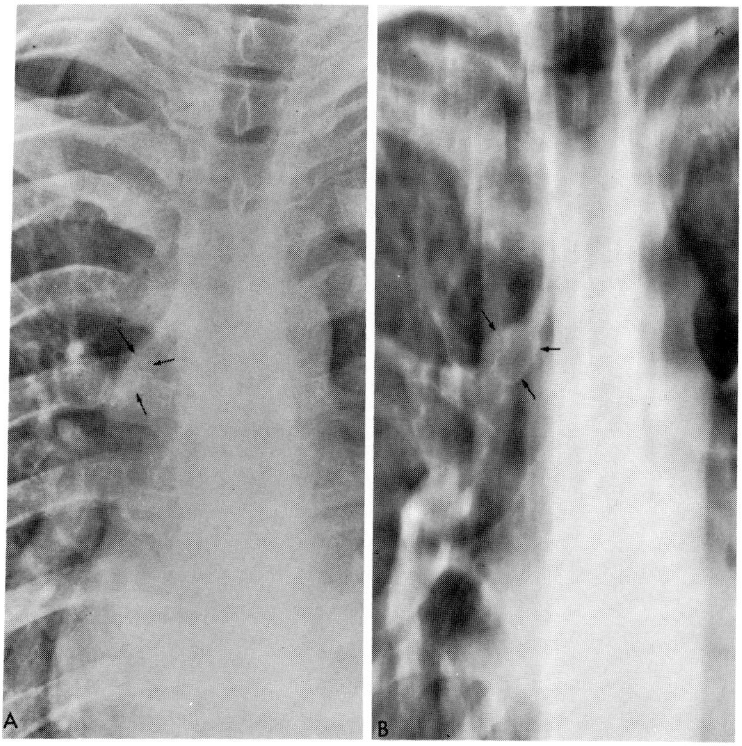

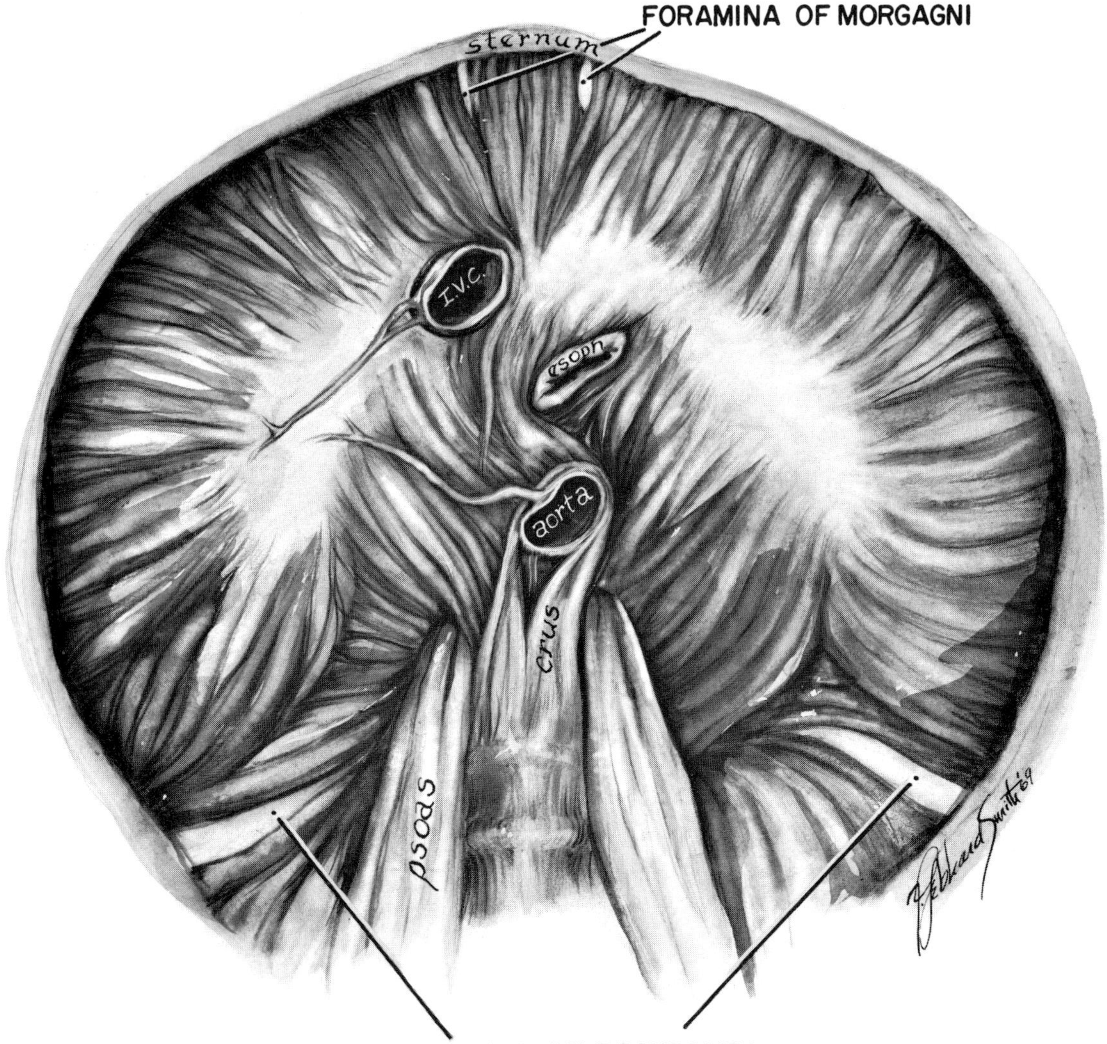

Figure 1–59A. Anatomy of the Normal Diaphragm Viewed from Below.

weight of 140 lb yielded a mean azygos-vein diameter of 14.2 mm; in only eight subjects was the weight-standardized vein diameter greater than 16 mm.

Visualization of this vein assumes considerable importance in some diseases, notably portal hypertension, obstruction of the superior vena cava, and congestive heart failure; familiarity with its normal roentgenographic appearance is important.

THE DIAPHRAGM

The diaphragm is a musculotendinous sheet which separates the thoracic cavity from the abdominal cavity (*see* Figure 1–59A). The central tendon is a broad sheet of decussating tendon fibers, in shape similar to a broad-bladed Australian boomerang; the point of the "boomerang" is directed toward the sternum and the concavity toward the spine. The muscle fibers arise anteriorly from the xiphoid process, around the convexity of the thorax from ribs seven to 12, posteriorly from the lateral margins of the first, second, and third lumbar vertebrae on the right side, and from the first and second lumbar vertebrae on the left. These fibers converge toward the central tendon and are inserted into it nearly perpendicular to its margin. The muscle fibers are of variable length, from 5 cm anteriorly at the sternal origin to 14 cm posterolaterally where they originate from the ninth, tenth, and eleventh ribs.[15] Von Hayek[15] points out that it is the posterolateral portion of the hemidiaphragms, where the muscle fibers are longest, that undergoes the greatest excursion on respiration. The muscle fibers which comprise the sternal attachment and those that arise from the seventh rib are separated bilaterally by triangular spaces poor in muscular and tendinous tissue. These triangular spaces, called the foramina of Morgagni, constitute weak areas in the diaphragm. Deficiencies in the origins of the muscle bundles from the posterolateral rib cage, called the foramina of Bochdalek, similarly create areas of potential weakness.

Roentgenographic Height of the Normal Diaphragm

Definitive study of the height of the hemidiaphragms on roentgenograms of normal adults was reported by Lennon and Simon[143] in 1965. These authors assessed frontal roentgenograms of the chest of 500 normal adults, 250 of each sex, all over 21 years of age. In 94 per cent, the level of the cupola of the right hemidiaphragm was projected in a plane ranging from the anterior end of the fifth rib to the sixth anterior interspace; 41 per cent were at the level of the sixth rib anteriorly; and only 4 per cent were at or below the level of the seventh rib. Generally speaking, the height of the right dome was higher in women, in subjects of heavy build, and in those over the age of 40.

Relationship Between the Height of the Right and Left Hemidiaphragms

The tendency for the right diaphragmatic dome to be on a plane approximately one-half an interspace higher than the left is well recognized, but of 500 normal subjects examined by Felson[69] the left hemidiaphragm was at the same height or was higher than the right in 9 per cent. Half the subjects comprising the 9 per cent had gaseous distension of the stomach or colon, a finding also mentioned by Simon[122] as being a common cause of left hemidiaphragmatic elevation. In 2 per cent of Felson's 500 cases the right hemidiaphragm was higher than the left by more than 3 cm.

It is a common error for students of roentgenology to ascribe elevation of the right hemidiaphragm to the presence of the mass of the liver beneath it. To these and other interested readers we recommend Wittenborg and Aviad's report[144] of their investigation of organ influence on normal diaphragmatic posture. These workers studied the chest roentgenograms of 60 children with anomalous organ positions. They found that the apex of the heart normally lies on the same side as the lower hemidiaphragm and that this relationship is maintained in the majority of cases of congenital malpositions of thoracic and abdominal viscera; further, they observed that the greater the degree of normality in development of the heart into a right and left side, the more often was the disparity in the height of the hemidiaphragms clearly defined and constant. The relationship of diaphragmatic height to cardiac anomalies is stated as follows: "In the presence of clear-cut inequalities in height of the hemidiaphragms (and absence of complicating pulmonary or neuromuscular disease) the odd-shaped cardiac silhouette may take on more meaning with the knowledge that, in all probability, the apex of the systemic or functional left ventricle is projected over the lower hemidiaphragm, irrespective of whether it be right or left and irrespective of the presence of anomalous positions of other organs."[144]

Thus it is clear that the lower position of one hemidiaphragmatic dome is intimately related to the presence of the contiguous mass of the left side of the heart.

Range of Diaphragmatic Excursion on Respiration

In a series of 204 patients studied by Simon,[161] the range of excursion of the two hemidiaphragms from full inspiration to full expiration was compared. In 23 per cent excursion was equal and symmetrical, in 50 per cent the right hemidiaphragm made a greater excursion than the left (mean difference, 0.75 cm), and the reverse occurred in 27 per cent (mean difference, 0.94 cm). In 188 patients, the mean excursion measured 3 to 6 cm in 140 (74 per cent), less than 3 cm in 44 (23 per cent), and greater than 6 cm in only four patients.

Physiologic Variations in Diaphragmatic Contour

Scalloping of the diaphragm, in which the normally smooth contour is replaced

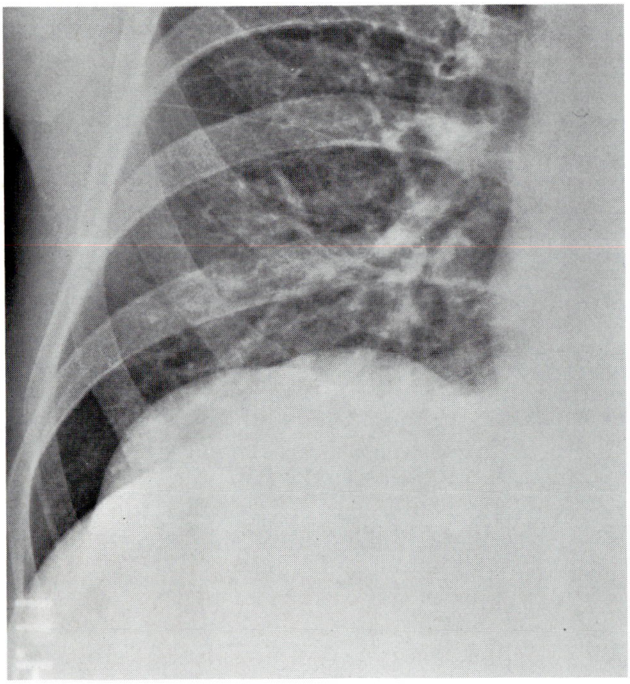

Figure 1–59B. **Scalloping of the Diaphragm.** A roentgenogram of the right hemidiaphragm reveals two smooth arcuate elevations disturbing the normally smooth contour of the dome, a finding of no known significance.

by a series of smooth arcuate elevations, is relatively uncommon (Figure 1–59*B*); Felson[69] observed it in only 5.5 per cent of 500 normal subjects. In the majority it was confined to the right side and in only a small percentage was it bilateral. The significance of this pattern is not known.

In some subjects, muscle slips originating from the lateral and posterolateral ribs may be visualized as short meniscus-shaped shadows along the lateral half of the hemidiaphragms bilaterally. These are produced by exceptionally low descent of the diaphragm during inspiration. Although such appearances are more common in association with severe pulmonary overinflation (Figure 1–60), as in asthma or emphysema, they may occur in the normal state, particularly in healthy young men; in the absence of supportive evidence they should not be interpreted as a sign of air-trapping.

Local "eventration" may occur anywhere in the diaphragm but is seen most commonly in the anteromedial quadrant on the right. This finding possesses no known significance.

THE CHEST WALL

The structures of the thoracic wall, both soft-tissue and osseous, form a complex of shadows on roentgenograms of the chest which may be important to roentgenographic analysis, and a working knowledge of their normal anatomy and variations is indispensable.

The Soft Tissues

On frontal roentgenograms of the thorax (*see* Figure 1–67, page 92) the soft tissues, consisting of the skin, subcutaneous fat, and muscles, usually are distinguishable along the upper shoulders and lateral thoracic wall, and on successive examinations may constitute a valuable sign of loss or gain in weight. The pectoral muscles form the anterior axillary fold, a structure which normally is visible in both male and female patients, curving smoothly downward and medially from the axilla to the rib cage. In men, particularly those with heavy muscular development, the inferior border of the pectoralis major muscle may be seen as a downward extension of the anterior axillary fold, passing obliquely across the middle portion of the lung fields bilaterally. In women, this shadow is obscured by the breasts, whose presence and size must be taken into consideration in assessment of density of the lower lung fields. Congenital absence of the pectoralis muscle occurs but is rare.[184]

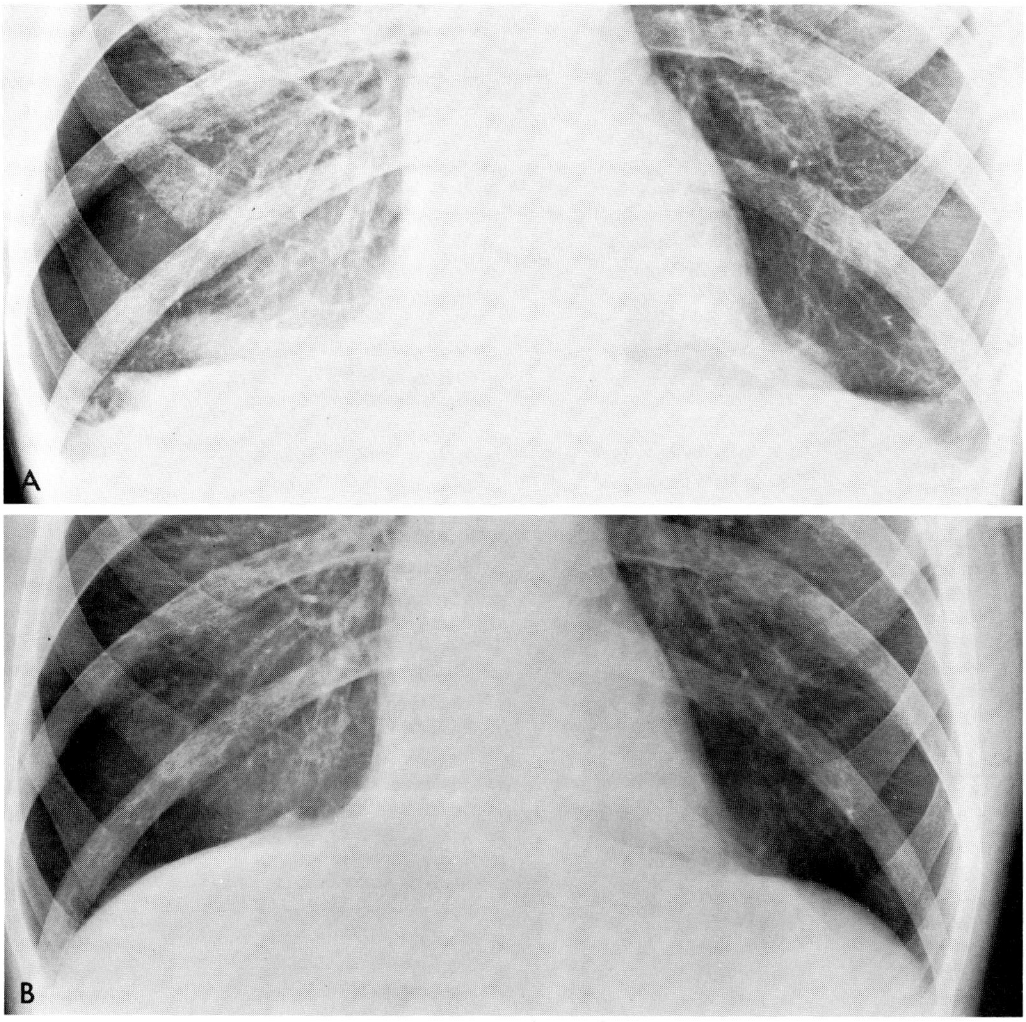

Figure 1–60. **Diaphragmatic Muscle Slips.** Inspiratory (*A*) and expiratory (*B*) roentgenograms of the lower half of the thorax of a patient with severe emphysema reveal short meniscus-shaped shadows extending laterally from each hemidiaphragm. These muscle slips are prominent on full inspiration and disappear on expiration.

In many cases the shadow of the sternomastoid muscle is visible as a density whose lateral margin parallels the spine in the medial third of the lung apices; it curves downward and laterally to blend with the companion shadow on the superior aspect of each clavicle. The latter shadow, which is 2 to 3 mm thick, parallels the superior aspect of the clavicle; it is formed by the skin and subcutaneous tissue overlying the clavicles and is rendered visible roentgenologically by the presence of the supraclavicular fossae and the tangential direction in which the x-ray beam strikes the clavicles.

Situated immediately behind the sternum is a structure to which little attention has been paid in the roentgenologic literature—the internal thoracic muscle.[146, 187] This muscle arises from the sternum, along the posteroinferior surface of the body and xiphoid, and extends upward and laterally to insert on the inner surfaces of the second through the sixth costal cartilages and adjacent ribs. In a series of 120 consecutive lateral chest roentgenograms, the muscle was identified as an obliquely placed density lying more or less parallel to the sternum in 37 patients, 26 male and 11 female.[146] In a more extensive roentgenographic study of 500 patients carried out by Shopfner and his colleagues,[187] the muscle was visualized in 390 (78 per cent).

The Bones

In the absence of pulmonary or pleural disease, deformity of the spine, or congen-

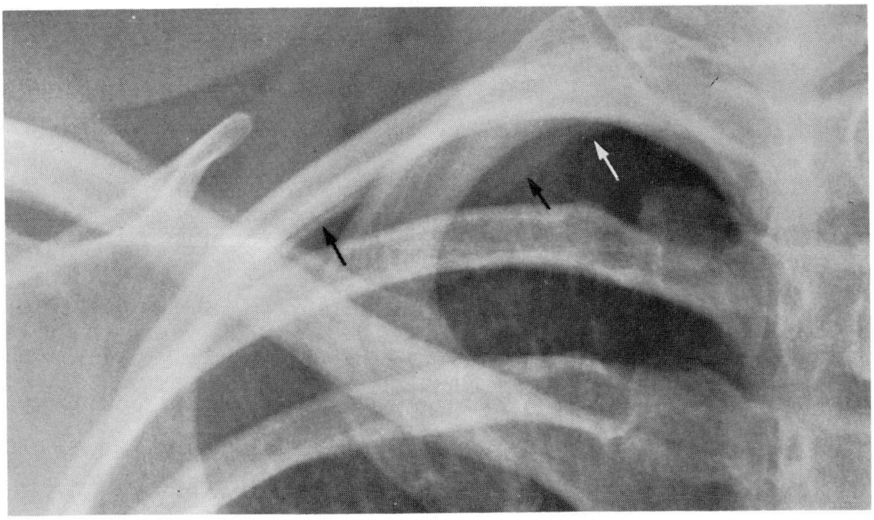

Figure 1–61. **Companion Shadows of the Ribs.** A magnified view of the apex of the right hemithorax reveals thin smooth shadows of water density lying roughly parallel to the inferior surfaces of the first and second ribs (arrows). These companion shadows are caused by visualization in tangential projection of a combination of parietal pleura and the soft tissues immediately external to the pleura.

ital anomalies of the ribs themselves, the rib cage should be perfectly symmetrical on the two sides. Both the upper and lower borders of the ribs should be sharply defined except in the middle and lower thoracic regions; here the thin flanges created by the vascular sulci on the inferior aspects of the ribs posteriorly are visualized *en face*, thus creating a less distinct inferior margin. In some cases the inferior aspects of the ribs posteriorly within 2 or 3 cm of their tubercles may show local superficial indentations; these should not be mistaken for pathologic rib notching, which is situated more laterally near the midclavicular line in cases of increased collateral circulation through the intercostal vessels.

Calcification of the rib cartilages occurs commonly, and probably is never of pathologic significance. The first-rib cartilage usually is the first to calcify, frequently shortly after the age of 20. In a roentgenographic study of 100 adults, 60 of whom were male and 40 female, Sanders[188] observed fairly consistent differences in the pattern of costal calcification in the two sexes: in the male, the upper and lower borders of the cartilage become calcified first, extending in continuity with the end of the rib; calcification of the central area follows. In contrast, calcification in women tends to occur first in a central location, in the form of either a solid tongue or as two parallel lines extending into the cartilage from the end of the rib. All of the five women who showed a "male pattern" of calcification had had previous pelvic surgery, and the author suggests that the pattern of costal cartilage calcification is under hormonal control.

Thin smooth shadows of water-density which parallel the ribs and measure 1 to 2 mm in diameter project adjacent to the inferior and inferolateral margins of the first and second ribs and to the axillary portions of the lower ribs. These "companion shadows" (Figure 1–61) are caused by visualization in tangential projection of a combination of parietal pleura and the soft tissues immediately external to the pleura; care must be taken not to misinterpret them as local pleural thickening. In 300 normal subjects in whom the companion shadows were specifically sought by Felson,[69] they were seen adjacent to the first rib in 35 per cent and the second rib in 31 per cent. In approximately half of the cases the shadows were bilateral; when unilateral, they were more commonly on the right side. Companion shadows adjacent to the axillary portions of the lower ribs were seen more often (in 75 per cent of 700 normal subjects).

Congenital anomalies of the ribs are relatively uncommon; supernumerary ribs (Figure 1–62) arising from the seventh cervical vertebra were identified in 1.5 per cent of 350 normal subjects examined by Felson;[69] nearly all were bilateral but many

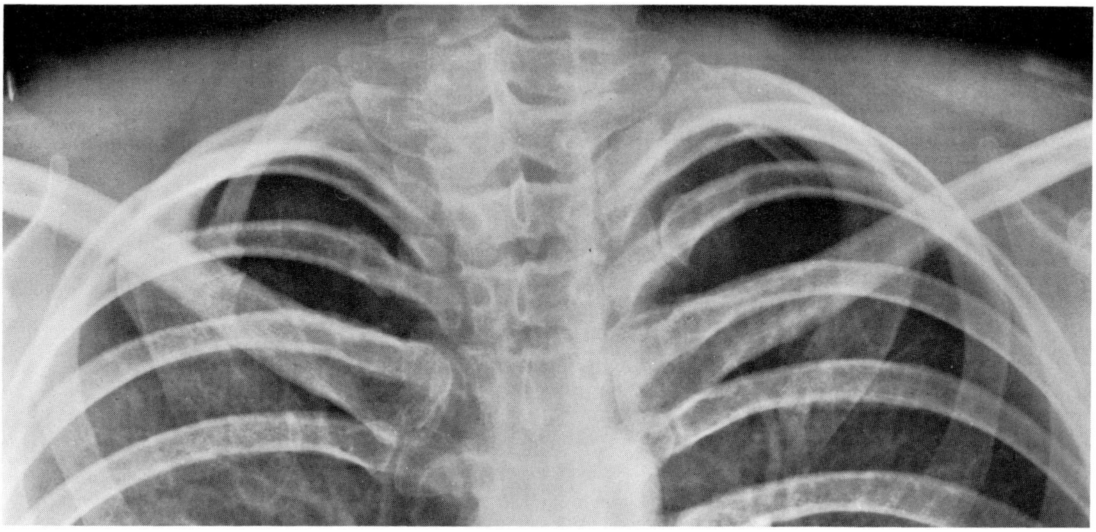

Figure 1–62. **Cervical Ribs.** Bilateral supernumerary ribs arise from the seventh cervical vertebra. The right rib is longer than the left and shows a synchondrosis with the medial aspect of the first rib.

had developed asymmetrically. Other anomalies, such as hypoplasia of the first rib (observed by Felson in 1.2 per cent of 350 normal subjects[69]), bifid or splayed anterior ribs, and, rarely, local fusion of ribs usually are important only in that they may result in an erroneous interpretation of abnormal lung density.

Occasionally the inferior aspect of the clavicles has an irregular notch or indentation 2 to 3 cm from the sternal articulation; this is of variable size and shape, from a superficial saucer-shaped defect to a deep notch 2 cm wide by 1.0 to 1.5 cm deep. These *rhomboid fossae* (Figure 1–63) give origin to the costoclavicular or rhomboid ligaments which radiate downward to bind the clavicle to the first rib.[145,184] The incidence varies from 10 per cent of clavicles studied anatomically[185] to 0.59 per cent of 10,000 photofluorograms reported by Shauffer and Collins.[186] Of the latter cases, 39 were unilateral and 20 bilateral.

A tiny foramen may be seen occasionally near the superior aspect of the center of the clavicle, either unilaterally or bilaterally; this foramen transmits the middle supraclavicular nerve and is said to be present in 6 per cent of dry skeletal specimens.[184]

The normal *thoracic spine* is perfectly straight in frontal projection and gently concave anteriorly in lateral projection. Its roentgenographic density in lateral projection decreases uniformly and progressively from above downward, and any deviation from this should arouse suspicion of intrathoracic disease.

The lateral and superior borders of the *manubrium* are the only portions of the sternum visible on frontal projections of

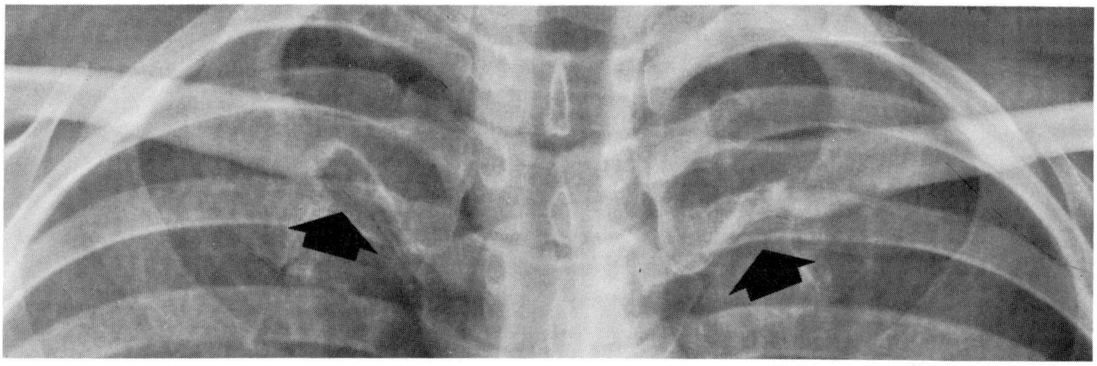

Figure 1–63. **Rhomboid Fossae.** An irregular notch or indentation is present in the inferior aspect of both clavicles approximately 2 cm from their sternal end (arrows). These fossae give origin to the costoclavicular or rhomboid ligaments

the thorax, although the whole of the sternum should be well visualized tangentially in lateral roentgenograms. Brief mention may be made of the intrathoracic rib, a rare congenital anomaly of which only ten examples had been reported by 1965.[147] This unusual anomaly consists of an accessory rib which arises within the bony thorax, more commonly on the right than the left, either from the anterior surface of a rib or from the contiguous vertebral body; it extends downward and slightly laterally to end at the diaphragm. Its only importance lies in its recognition as an innocuous intrathoracic structure.

THE NORMAL CHEST ROENTGENOGRAM

As the preceding sections have shown, the lungs are composed of an almost incredible complex of tissues, each of which separately performs a unique function but all of which, when integrated, perform the act of respiration. The morphologist can examine each tissue and pronounce on its normal or abnormal characteristics; in many ways, through the application of special techniques such as bronchography and angiography, the roentgenologist may similarly assess individual components of the lungs, although his methods are necessarily more gross in scope. However, the bulk of roentgenograms of the chest which the diagnostician must interpret are plain films, with no help from contrast media, and here he is dealing with a summation of relatively low-contrast objects forming a complex group of roentgenographic shadows of varying definition and density. The composition of the lungs in relation to their "density"* and to their roentgenographic pattern is a facet of chest roentgenology which has received insufficient attention in the literature, and in this section an attempt is made to clarify some of these issues.

*In this context, the word "density" applies to the *weight of tissue per volume*, or specific gravity (for comparative purposes, the figures for lung tissue may be related to the density of soft tissue as equivalent to water at 1.0 g per ml and to the density of air as zero). It should not be confused with "roentgenographic density," which is a measure of the blackening of film caused by a reduction in silver emulsion by the incident roentgen beam. The greater the amount of radiation which passes through the body, the greater will be the blackening of the roentgenogram; thus, since the tissue density of bone is greater than that of lung, transmission of roentgen rays through bone is less, so that on chest roentgenograms bones appear relatively white in comparison with the blackness of lung. Therefore, *roentgenographic density is dependent upon "tissue" density*, at least in adequately exposed chest roentgenograms.

Table 1–4. Pulmonary Tissue and Blood Volumes in ml

	EXTRAVASCULAR TISSUE VOLUME	PULMONARY BLOOD VOLUME	TOTAL MAXIMAL TISSUE VOLUME
Staub,[22] 1963*	275	350	625
Loyd, *et al.*,[149] 1966†	420	430	850
Average	350	390	740

*Estimate of the lungs of a 70 kg man, based on anatomic studies of five healthy men.

†Estimate of the lungs of a 70 kg man, 70 inches in height, derived from a nomogram constructed by Loyd and his associates[149] from physiologic data (based on the determination of pulmonary tissue volume described by Sackner and his co-workers[150] and of pulmonary blood volume described by McGaff and his associates[151]).

Normal Lung Density

It is readily apparent that the "roentgenographic density" of the lungs is the result of the absorptive powers of each of its component parts—gas, blood, and tissue. Although precise figures for the relative contributions of blood and tissue vary somewhat depending upon whether results are obtained by anatomic or physiologic methods, data have been compiled which allow a reasonable approximation (*see* Table 1–4).

If we apply the *average* figures for total maximal tissue volume, derived from anatomic and physiologic estimates, and the predicted total lung capacity (6500 ml)[152] of a 20-year-old man, 170 cm in height, the *average density* of lung is 740 g: 7240 ml,* or 0.10 g per ml.

This figure, of course, represents the density of a structure whose composite parts are uniformly distributed throughout it, a situation which hardly pertains in the lung. Some of the roentgenographic density of lung is contributed to by the major blood vessels, which are visible as homogeneous tapering structures having a density of 1.0 g per ml. Since the average density of lung is only 0.10, a considerable portion of lung tissue must possess a density *less* than this,

*The ratio of total weight (740 g, with a volume of 740 ml) to total volume (6500 ml + 740 ml).

to compensate for the relatively high density of the visible blood vessels; obviously a high proportion of air must be contained in such tissue—logically, the lung parenchyma or respiratory portion of the lung.

Weibel[81] estimated that the lung parenchyma comprises 90 per cent of total lung volume. By use of a point-counting technique, the same investigator measured the volumetric proportion of the three components of lung parenchyma: *air* accounted for 92 per cent, and *tissue and capillary blood*, 8.0 per cent (including interstitium, endothelial, and epithelial cells, vessel walls, and blood). On the basis of Weibel's figures and again assuming a total lung volume of 7240 ml, the parenchymal component is approximately 6500 ml (90 per cent of 7240 ml), of which 500 ml consists of tissue and blood (8 per cent of 6500 ml). Thus, *the density of lung parenchyma at total lung capacity is 0.08* (500 g: 6500 ml). *It follows that in a chest roentgenogram all the tissue visible in the peripheral 2 cm of the lung or between vascular shadows has a density of 0.08 g per ml.*

If the extravascular tissue volume is assumed to be constant, the overall roentgenographic density of lung (average, 0.1 g/ml) is the result of the ratio of its blood and gas content. The blood content may be further subdivided into a capillary component, which creates the *background density* of the lung parenchyma (0.08 g/ml), and a larger vessel component, which creates the *visible lung markings* (density, 1.0 g/ml). Figures for *total capillary blood volume* vary according to the technique used for measurement. Physiologic techniques have yielded estimates, in the resting subject, of 60 to 100 ml,[22, 77-79] whereas anatomic studies have indicated a volume of 150 to 200 ml.[81, 82] Piiper[202] subdivided total pulmonary blood volume in the dog into its three vascular components and estimated 27 per cent to be in the arteries, 38 per cent in capillaries, and 35 per cent in veins. If these percentages can be extended to the human lung, the average of 390 ml for total pulmonary blood volume (*see* Table 1–4) may be broken down to indicate a *capillary volume of 150 ml and a larger-vessel volume of 240 ml.* A capillary blood volume of 150 ml probably represents an acceptable average of the figures obtained by anatomic and physiologic techniques of measurement, although it is somewhat higher than the figures quoted earlier in this book in the discussion on physiology of acinar perfusion.

It is important to appreciate the distinction between capillary and visible vessel components of the lung, in their separate contributions to lung density. For example, variation in total *capillary* blood volume probably is difficult, if not impossible, to appreciate subjectively on plain roentgenograms of the chest (although this may be accomplished objectively by roentgen densitometry). Although an increase in capillary blood volume is known to occur in ventricular septal defect[154] and in atrial septal defect,[155] without concomitant alteration in lung volumes,[156] it is doubtful whether the increase in lung density which must result from this increased capillary volume can be appreciated roentgenographically, except by densitometric means. In such situations, roentgenologic assessment of vascular plethora (pleonemia) must be based on an increase in the size and number of visible pulmonary vessels, both arterial and venous.

It is emphasized that these statements apply only to conditions in which *uniform* alteration in perfusion exists throughout the lungs—for example, in the pleonemia that accompanies intracardiac left-to-right shunt (Figure 1–64*A*) or in the oligemia of diffuse emphysema (Figure 1–64*B*). When reduction in blood flow is local, as with lobar emphysema (Figure 1–64*C*) or occasionally with massive pulmonary embolism (Westermark's sign[157]), alteration in density in the involved area of lung is the result of a reduction in *both* capillary blood volume (background density) and visible vascular shadows. Such alteration of background lung density is an exceedingly valuable roentgenologic sign.

Alteration in Lung Density

In any clinical situation, alteration in roentgenographic lung density may be due to one of three mechanisms or a combination thereof.

PHYSIOLOGIC MECHANISMS. A frequently observed physiologic variation in lung density with which every roentgenologist is familiar is the change that may occur from one examination to another on the same subject, depending upon depth of inspiration. Such variation is readily explained by comparing the contributions of the three components of the lung to its density. For example, again consider a 20-year-old man, 170 cm in height, and assume that pulmonary blood volume and tissue volume are reasonably constant at different degrees

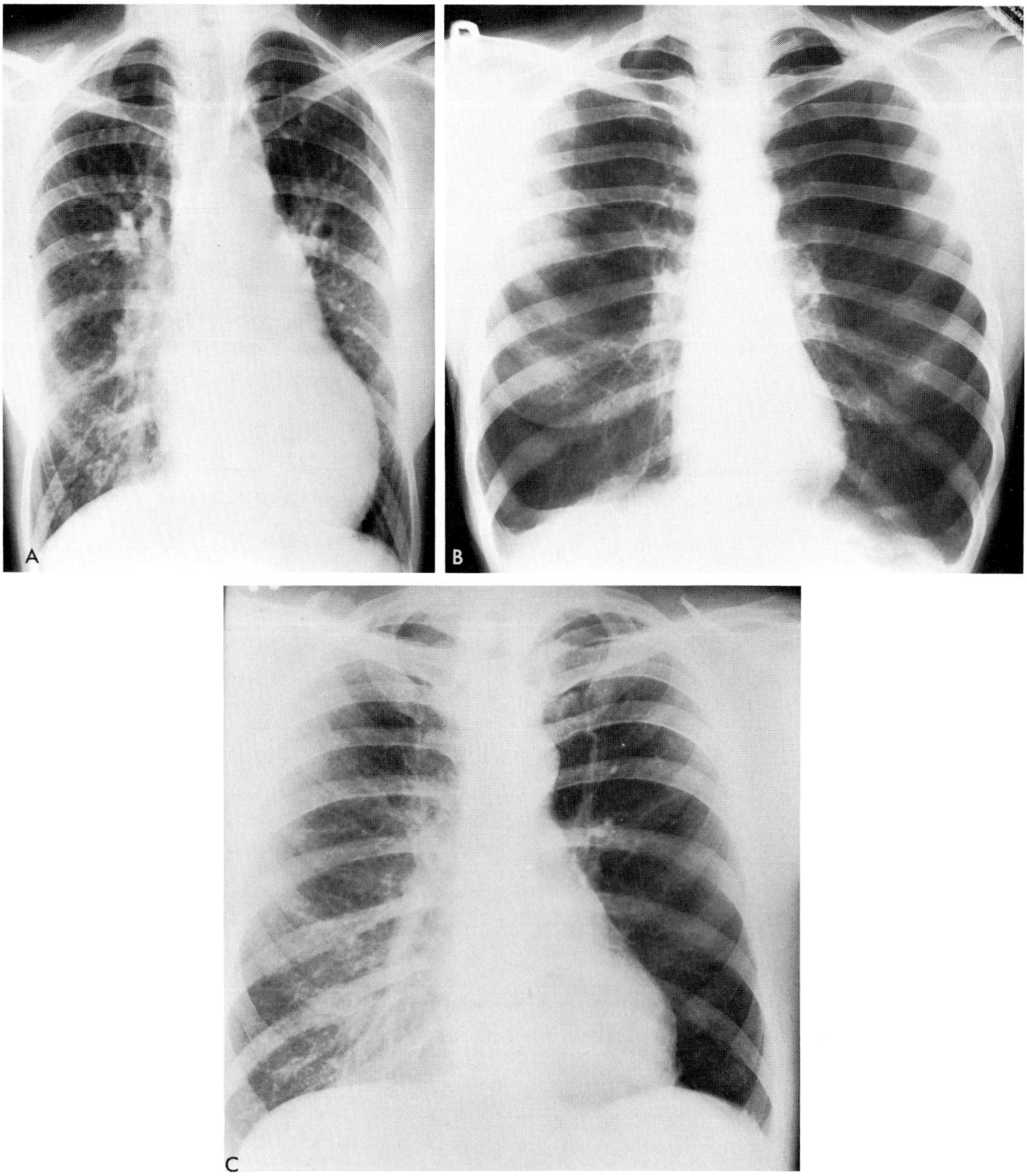

Figure 1–64. **Alteration in Lung Density Owing to Abnormalities of Perfusion.** Generalized pleonemia as seen in patent ductus arteriosus (*A*) and diffuse oligemia as in generalized emphysema (*B*) are evidenced by an increase or decrease, respectively, in the size of the major pulmonary vessels rather than by discernible alteration in background lung density. When alteration in blood flow is local as in unilateral emphysema (Swyer-James syndrome) (*C*), reduction in density is apparent because of a decrease in *both* capillary blood volume (background density) and visible vascular shadows.

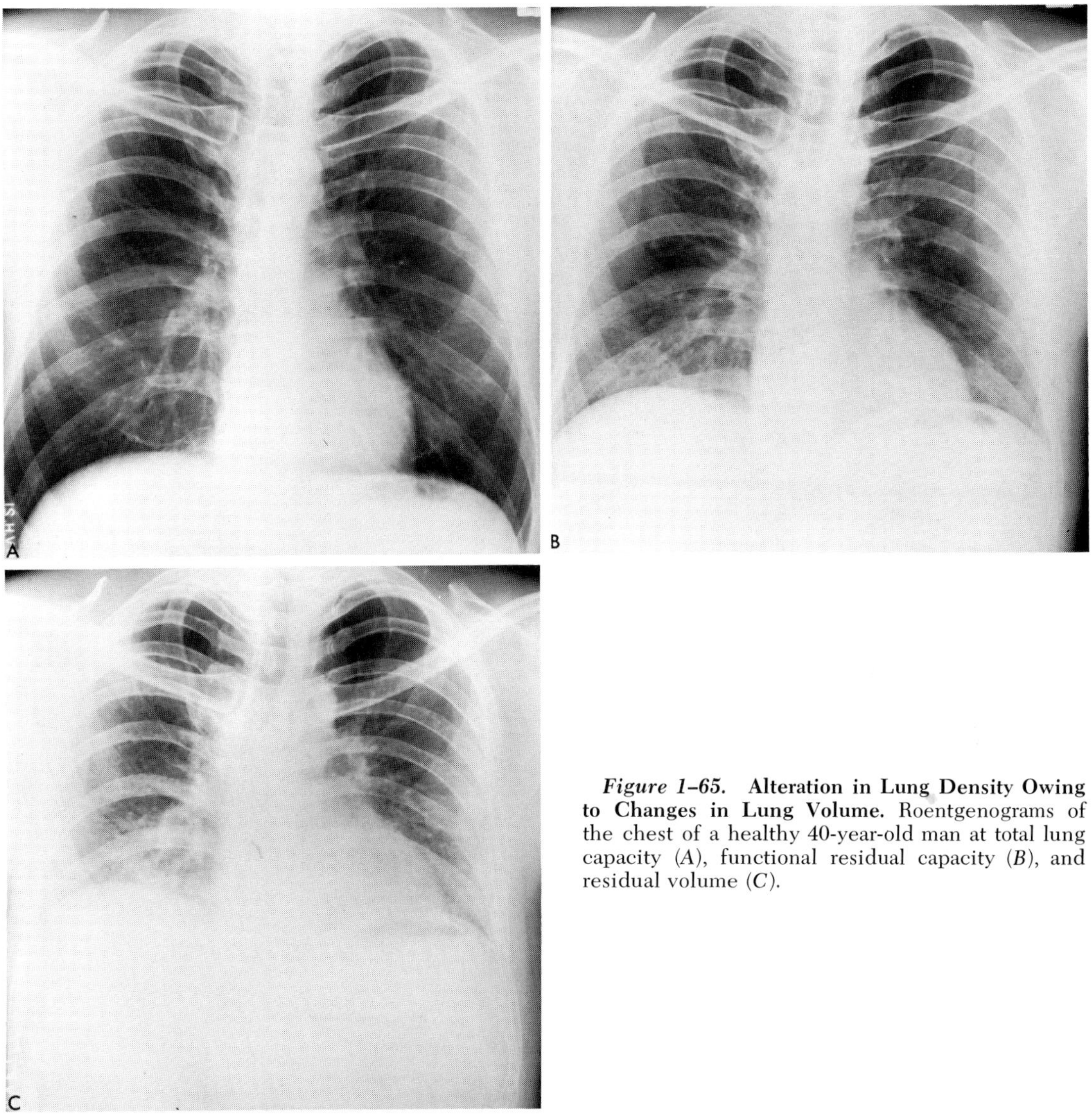

Figure 1–65. **Alteration in Lung Density Owing to Changes in Lung Volume.** Roentgenograms of the chest of a healthy 40-year-old man at total lung capacity (*A*), functional residual capacity (*B*), and residual volume (*C*).

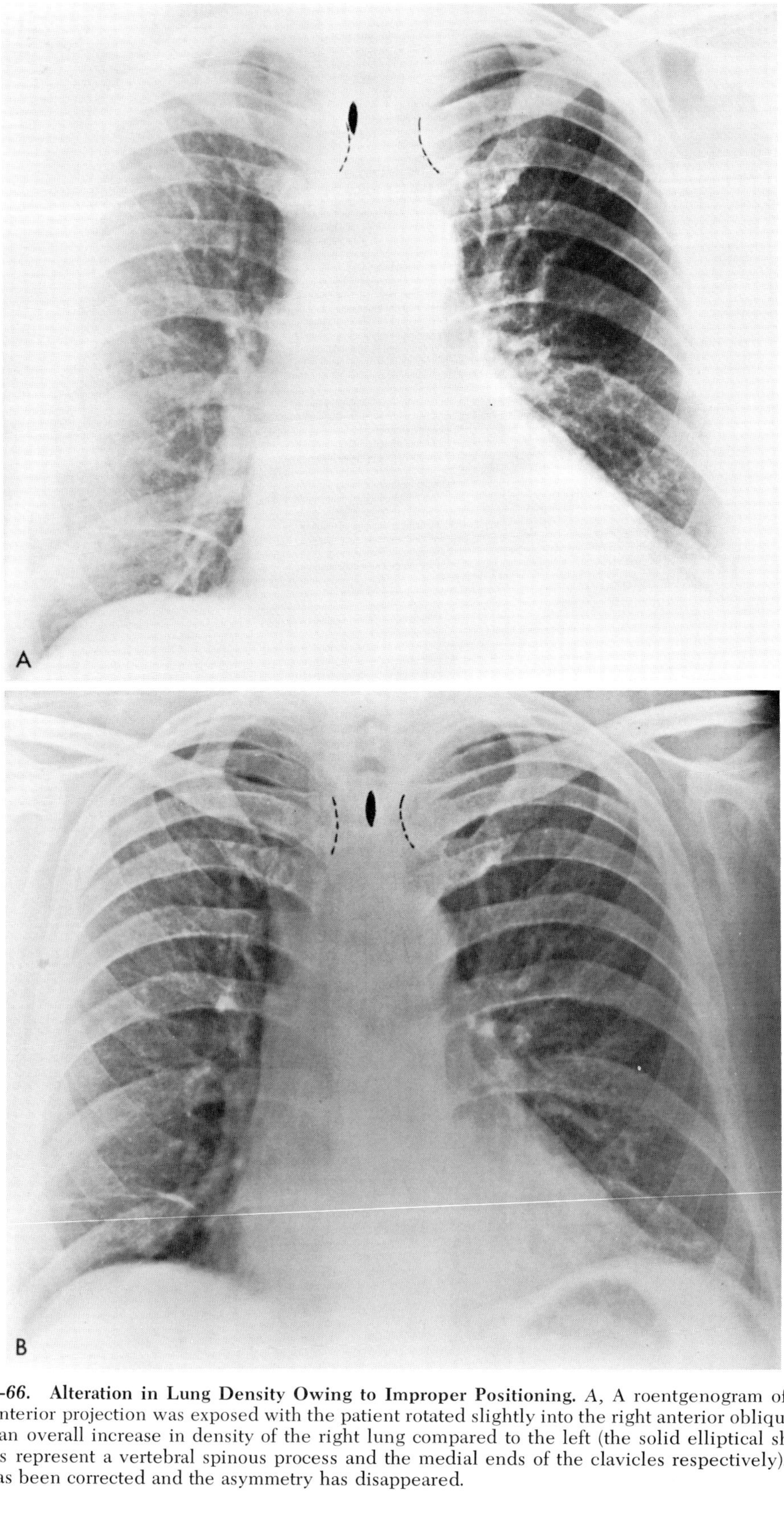

Figure 1–66. **Alteration in Lung Density Owing to Improper Positioning.** *A*, A roentgenogram of the chest in posteroanterior projection was exposed with the patient rotated slightly into the right anterior oblique position, producing an overall increase in density of the right lung compared to the left (the solid elliptical shadow and dotted lines represent a vertebral spinous process and the medial ends of the clavicles respectively). In *B*, positioning has been corrected and the asymmetry has disappeared.

Table 1–5. The Composition and Density of Normal Lung

LUNG VOLUME			
Arterial blood volume*	105 ml		
Capillary blood volume*	150 ml		
Venous blood volume*	135 ml		
Total pulmonary blood volume	390 ml†		
Extravascular tissue volume	350 ml†		
Total blood and tissue volume	740 ml		
Total lung capacity‡	6500 ml		
Total lung volume	7240 ml		
LUNG DENSITY			
Average density at TLC (6500 ml) = 7240/740		0.10 g/ml	
Average density at FRC (3400 ml) = 4140/740		0.18 g/ml	
Average density at RV (1500 ml) = 2240/740		0.33 g/ml	
PARENCHYMAL VOLUME			
Lung parenchyma = 90% total lung volume§ (90% 7240 ml)			6500 ml
Tissue and capillary blood (8% of parenchyma§)			500 ml
Air (92% of parenchyma§)			6000 ml
PARENCHYMAL DENSITY			
Density at TLC = 6500/500		0.08 g/ml	

*Piiper[202]
†*See* Table 1–4 (page 86)
‡20-year-old man 170 cm in height[152]
§Weibel,[81] 1962

of lung inflation; according to the tables of normal values constructed by Goldman and Becklake,[152] predicted lung volumes for such a subject will be: total lung capacity, 6.5 liters; functional residual capacity, 3.4 liters; and residual volume, 1.5 liters. Assuming a total maximal tissue volume of 740 ml, average lung density at total lung capacity is 0.10; at functional residual capacity, density is almost double (0.18), and at residual volume it is more than treble (0.33) (Figure 1–65). Thus, it is clear that, assuming total pulmonary blood volume to be constant at different degrees of lung inflation, *lung density is inversely proportional to the amount of contained gas.*

PHYSICAL (OR TECHNICAL) MECHANISMS. Symmetry of roentgenographic density of the two lungs in a normal subject is dependent upon proper positioning of the patient for roentgenography. If the patient is rotated as little as 2 to 3 degrees, the density of the lung closer to the film will be uniformly *greater* than the density of the other lung (Figure 1–66). This effect is produced by the greater thickness of thoracic-wall musculature through which the x-ray beam must pass when a patient is rotated either to the right or to the left. A similar effect may be produced by scoliosis or by incorrect centering of the x-ray beam. Since comparison of the density of the two lungs plays such an important part in the assessment of chest roentgenograms, correct positioning of the patient and centering of the x-ray beam are crucial.

PATHOLOGIC MECHANISMS. Excluding from consideration the contribution to roentgenographic density from the soft tissues of the thoracic wall and providing that physiologic and physical causes can be excluded, variation in lung density always is due to an increase or decrease in one or more of the three elements, air, blood, and tissue. A change in density is seldom produced by alteration in one component to the exclusion of the others: examples of such "pure" alteration are the reduction in density (increased translucency) produced by pulmonary embolism without infarction (Westermark's sign), in which there is reduction in blood volume but little change in gas or tissue volume; or diffuse pulmonary infiltration, such as sarcoidosis, in which there is increase in extravascular tissue volume but little change in gas or blood volume. In the majority of clinical situations, change in density, whether increased or decreased, local or diffuse, is the result of a change in all three components. The relative contribution of each component is discussed in detail in the appropriate sections.

In Table 1–5 is summarized the contributions to the total volume of the lungs of their component parts, together with the average density of lung at different vol-

(Text continued on page 97)

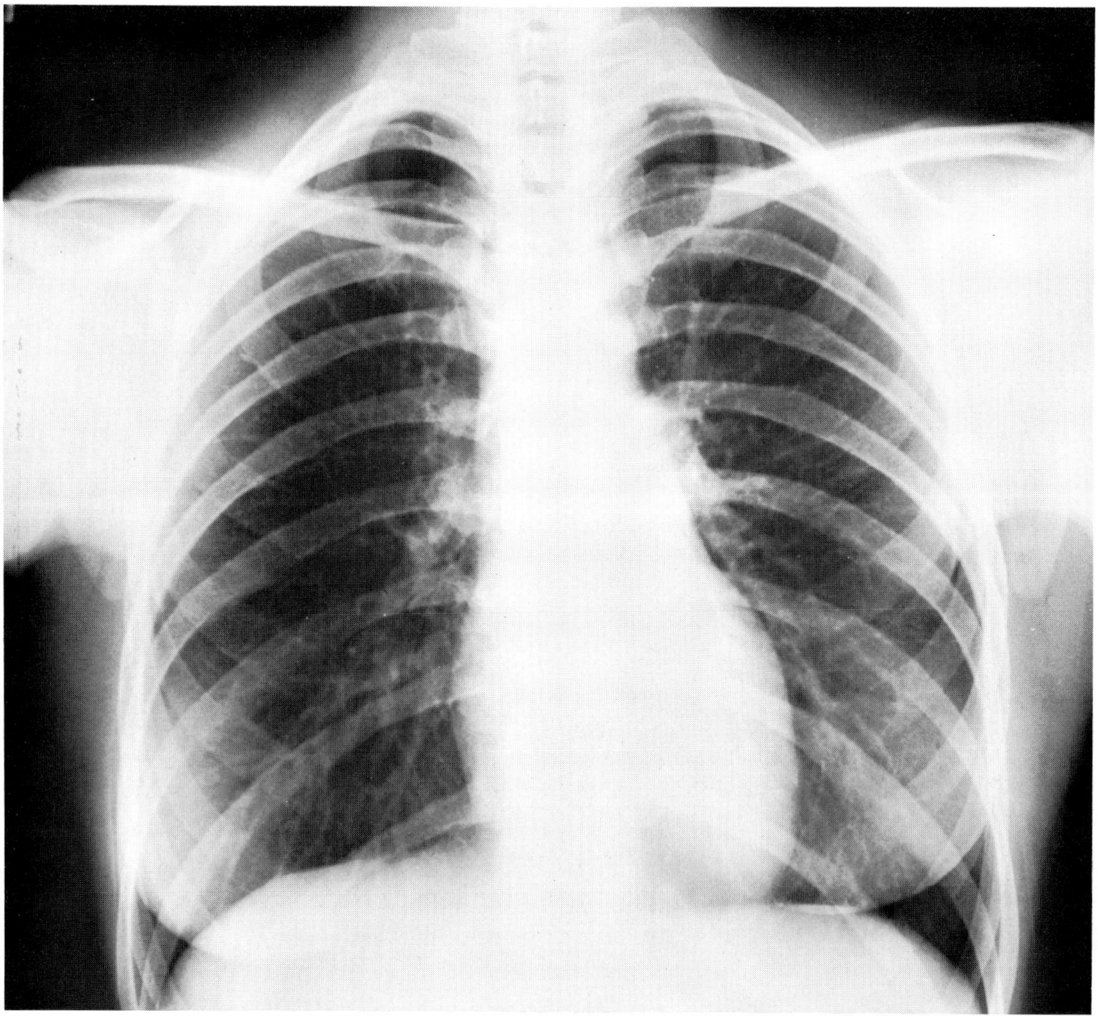

A

Figure 1–67. **Normal Chest Roentgenogram, Posteroanterior Projection.** *A*, A roentgenogram of the chest in the erect position of an asymptomatic 26-year-old woman.

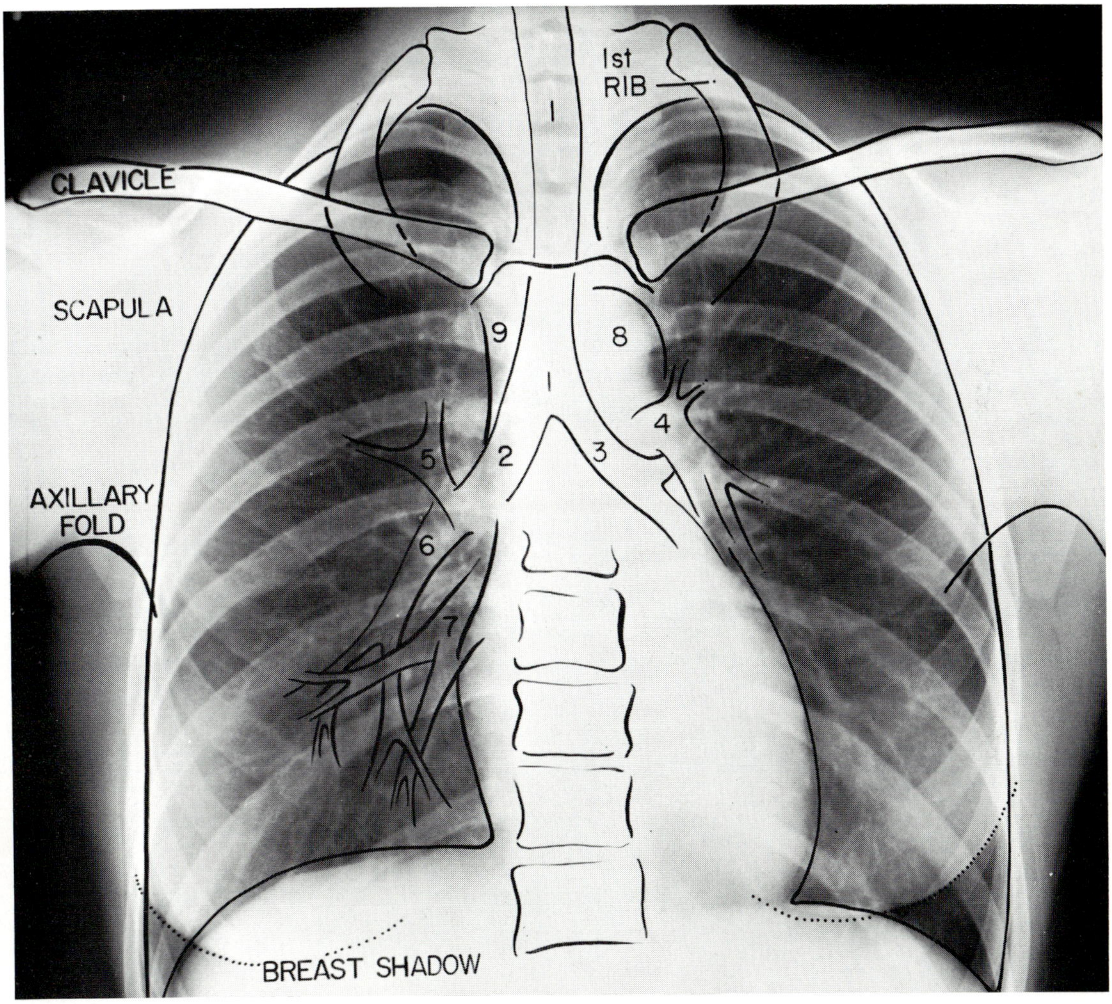

B

Figure 1–67. Continued. *B,* A diagrammatic overlay shows the normal anatomic structures numbered or labeled: (1) trachea; (2) right main bronchus; (3) left main bronchus; (4) left pulmonary artery; (5) right upper lobe pulmonary vein; (6) right interlobar artery; (7) right lower and middle lobe vein; (8) aortic knob; (9) superior vena cava.

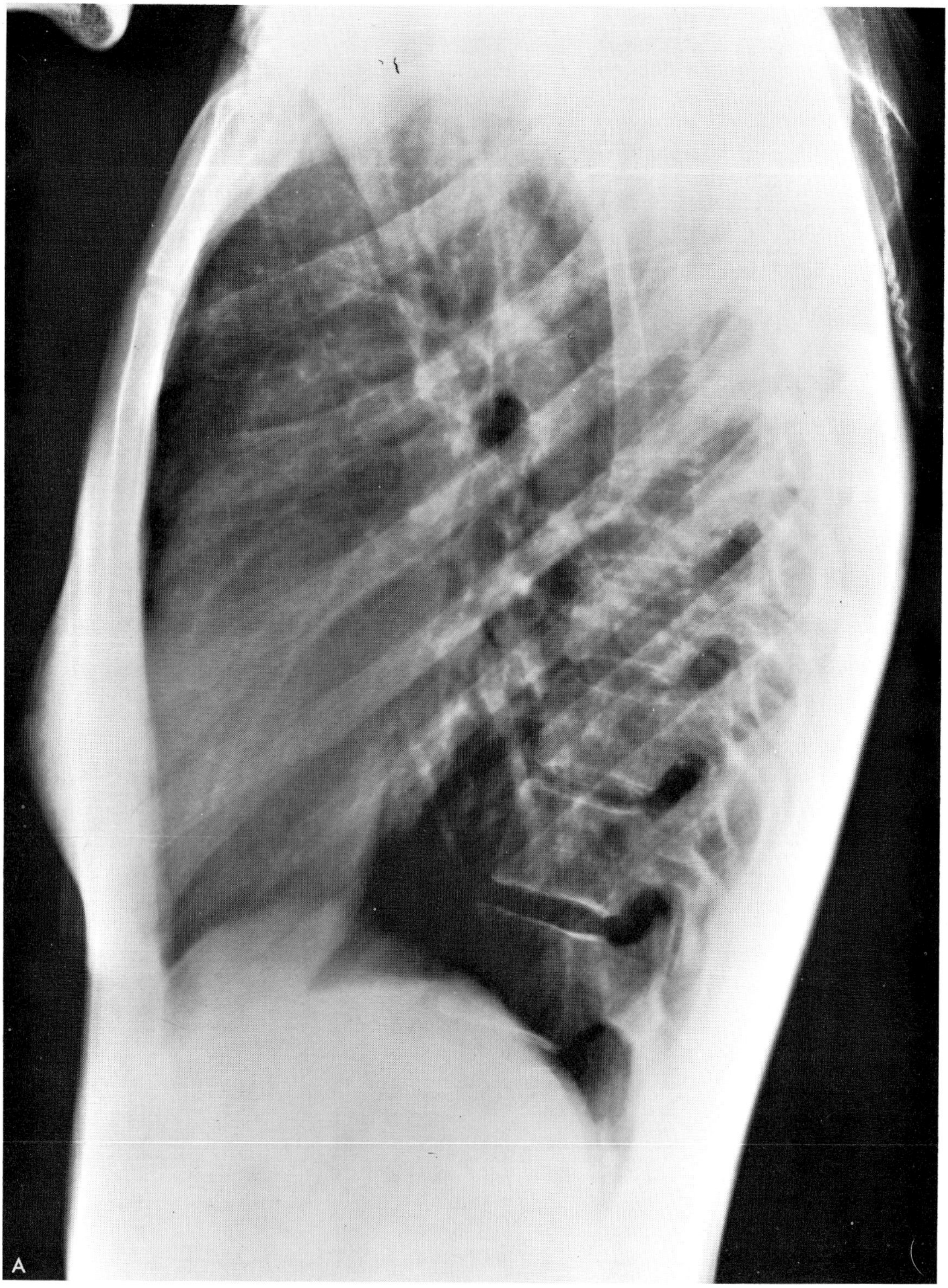

Figure 1–68. **Normal Chest Roentgenogram, Lateral Projection.** *A*, A roentgenogram of the chest in the erect position of an asymptomatic 26-year-old woman.

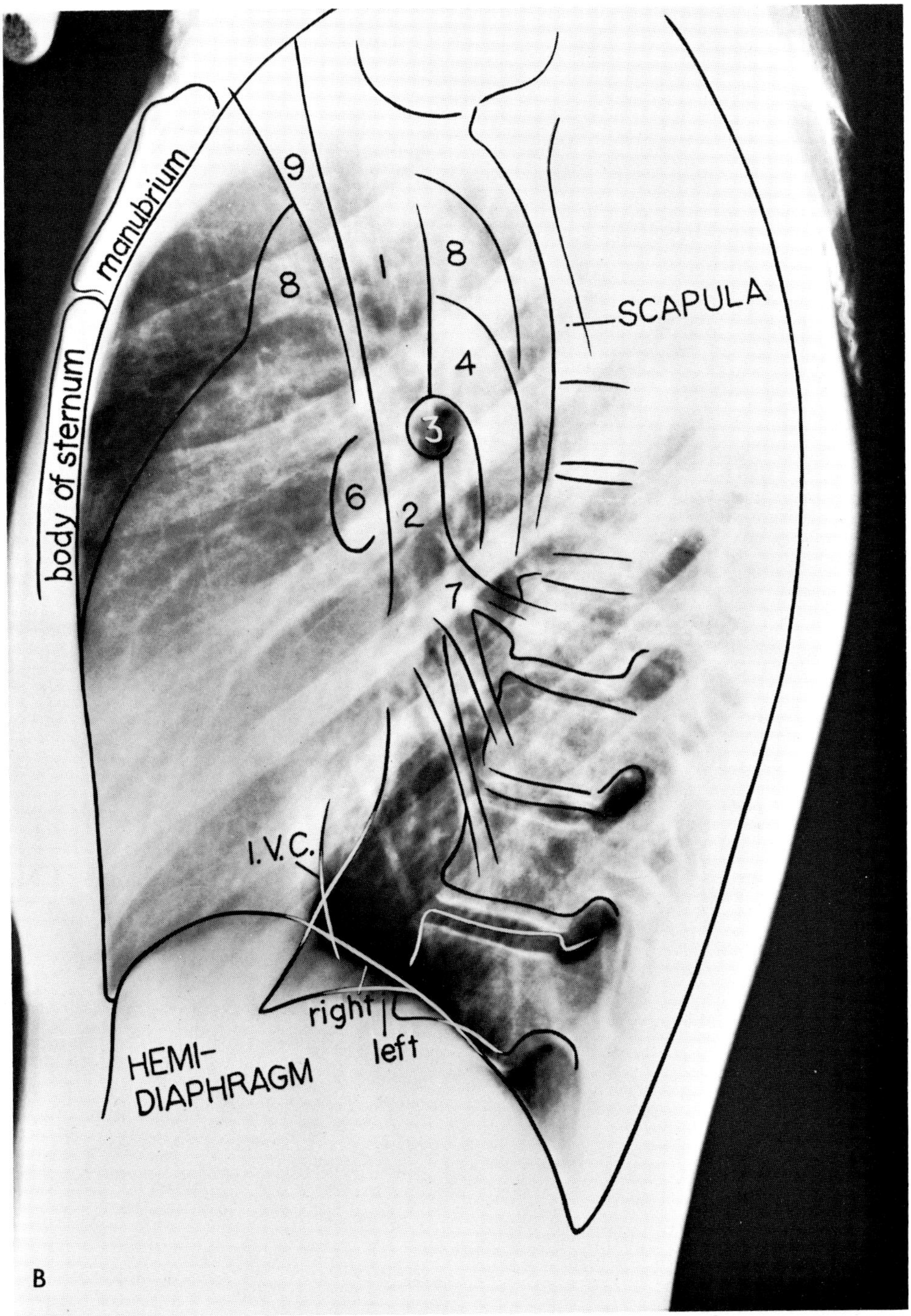

Figure 1–68. Continued. *B*, A diagrammatic overlay shows the normal anatomic structures numbered or labeled: (1) trachea; (2) right intermediate bronchus; (3) left upper lobe bronchus; (4) left interlobar artery; (6) right main pulmonary artery; (7) confluence of pulmonary veins; (8) aortic arch; (9) brachiocephalic vessels.

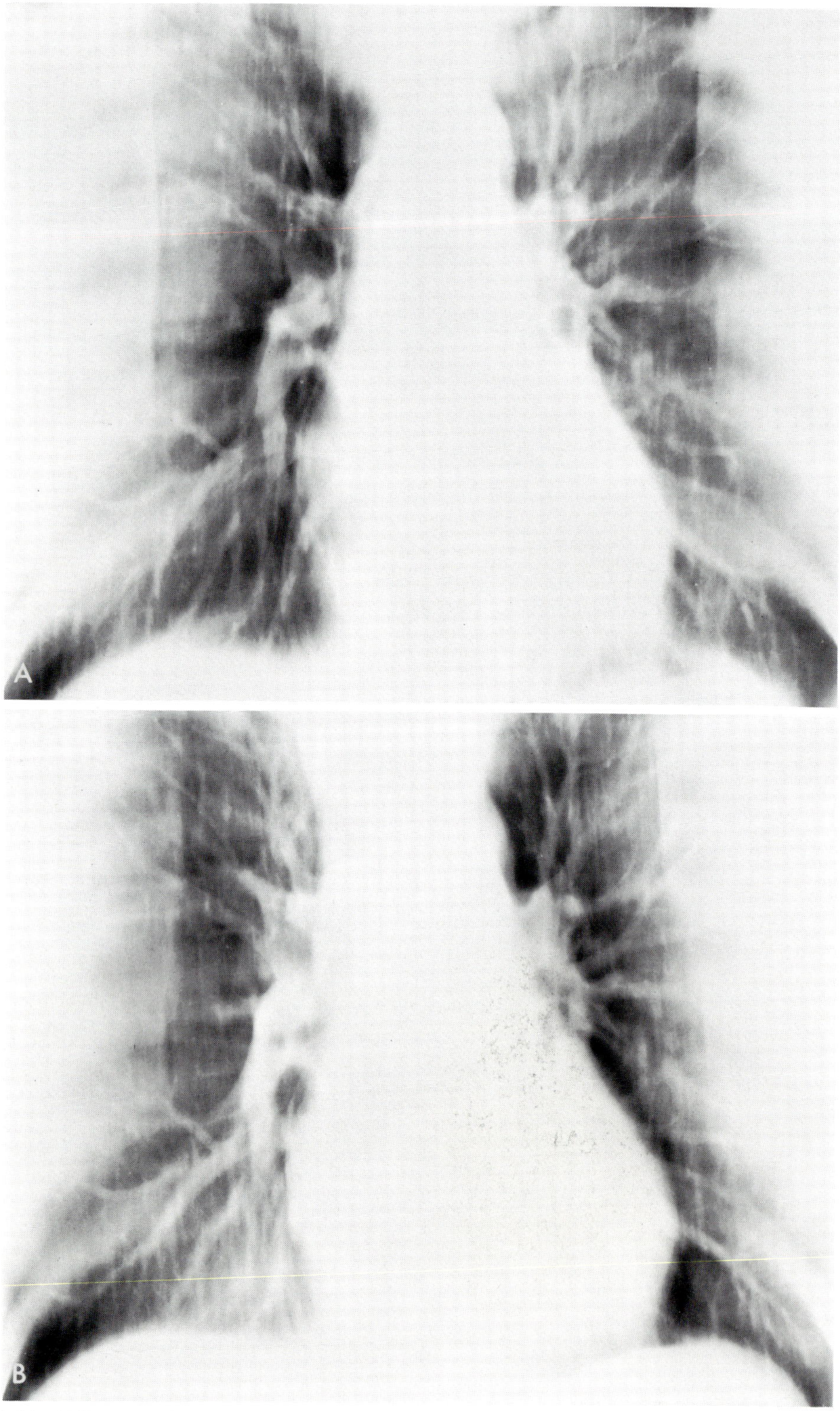

Figure 1–69. **Effect on Pulmonary Vasculature of Change in Body Position.** Tomographic sections through the midportion of both lungs in the erect (*A*) and supine (*B*) positions reveal a significant difference in the size of vascular channels. In the supine roentgenogram, not only are the upper lobe arteries and veins more prominent than in the erect study but the overall "grayness" of the upper zones is greater, indicating increased capillary perfusion. Note the difference in the size of the azygos vein in the two studies.

umes, and the composition and density of lung parenchyma.

The Pulmonary Markings

It is of the utmost importance for the roentgenologist to have a thorough knowledge of the pattern of linear markings throughout the normal lung. Unfortunately, such knowledge cannot be gained through didactic teaching; it requires exposure to thousands of normal chest roentgenograms to acquire the experience—perhaps, more, the art—to be able to distinguish normal from abnormal. It requires not only familiarity with the distribution and pattern of branching of these markings (which are described in the section on roentgen anatomy), but also an awareness of normal caliber, extent of normal roentgenologic visibility, and changes that may occur in different phases of respiration and in various body positions. There are two main reasons for the need of such knowledge: (1) a change in the caliber of arteries and veins constitutes one of the most valuable roentgenologic signs of pulmonary venous and pulmonary arterial hypertension and (2) a redistribution of vessels, with consequent modification of the number of roentgenologically visible markings, may constitute the major evidence for pulmonary collapse or previous pulmonary resection.

The linear markings are created by a complex bundle of structures which are intimately related to one another in their passage through the lungs (Figures 1–67 and 1–68). These structures are the pulmonary arteries, the bronchial arteries, the bronchi, the nerves, and the lymphatic channels and lymphoid collections; all of these structures are connected, at least proximal to the arterioles, by a cuff of loose areolar tissue. The arterial bundles fan outward from both hila, tapering gradually as they proceed distally. In the normal state they are visible to about 1 to 2 cm from the visceral pleural surface over the convexity of the lung, at which point lung structure becomes totally acinar in type and the lung markings invisible (the lung parenchyma). Jefferson[70] pointed out that on arteriograms a centimeter and millimeter pattern of branching vessels can be identified in the periphery of the lung, analogous to the pattern on bronchograms described by Reid and Simon;[158] only rarely, however, can such a pattern be distinguished on plain roentgenograms.

As is indicated in a previous section dealing with the pulmonary vascular tree, the anatomic remoteness of the pulmonary veins from the arteries often renders their distinction possible roentgenographically (*see* Figure 1–37, page 42). In the region of the pulmonary ligaments, especially, no difficulty should be encountered in distinguishing these vessels, since the pulmonary veins in the lower lung zones lie almost horizontally and on a lower plane than the arteries (*see* Figure 1–36, page 40). Simon[162] pointed out that a horizontal line drawn across a posteroanterior roentgenogram of the chest at a midpoint between the apex and diaphragm separates the pulmonary artery complex in the hila (at or above this line) and the veins (below the line). The veins which drain the upper lobes are lateral to their respective arteries, not only in the hilar regions but in the lung fields also. This relationship is particularly valuable in the right hilar region, where the superior pulmonary vein forms the lateral aspect of the hilum superiorly and thus produces the upper limb of its concave configuration (*see* Figure 1–37). Flattening of this concavity provides good evidence for collapse of the right upper lobe, or, in the presence of pulmonary venous hypertension, indicates engorgement of the upper-lobe vein.[159]

In a roentgenogram of the chest of an erect subject there is usually some discrepancy between the size of the linear markings in the upper lung fields compared with those in the lower, due largely to lesser perfusion of the upper zones. Because of hydrostatic pressure, when the subject is erect, pulmonary blood flow increases progressively from apex to base, a unit volume of lung at the base of the thorax having four to eight times the blood flow of a similar volume at the apex.[104] When roentgenography is carried out with the patient in the horizontal position, this discrepancy in vascular size largely disappears, due to removal of the influence of gravity. The caliber of the upper-lobe vessels in such circumstances is influenced also by the increase in pulmonary blood volume which occurs when the patient is supine and which, according to Daley and his associates, amounts to approximately 30 per cent.[160] Thus, the gravitational advantage enjoyed by the upper lobes in the supine position may result in the upper-lobe vasculature appearing quite different in such films compared with films made in the erect

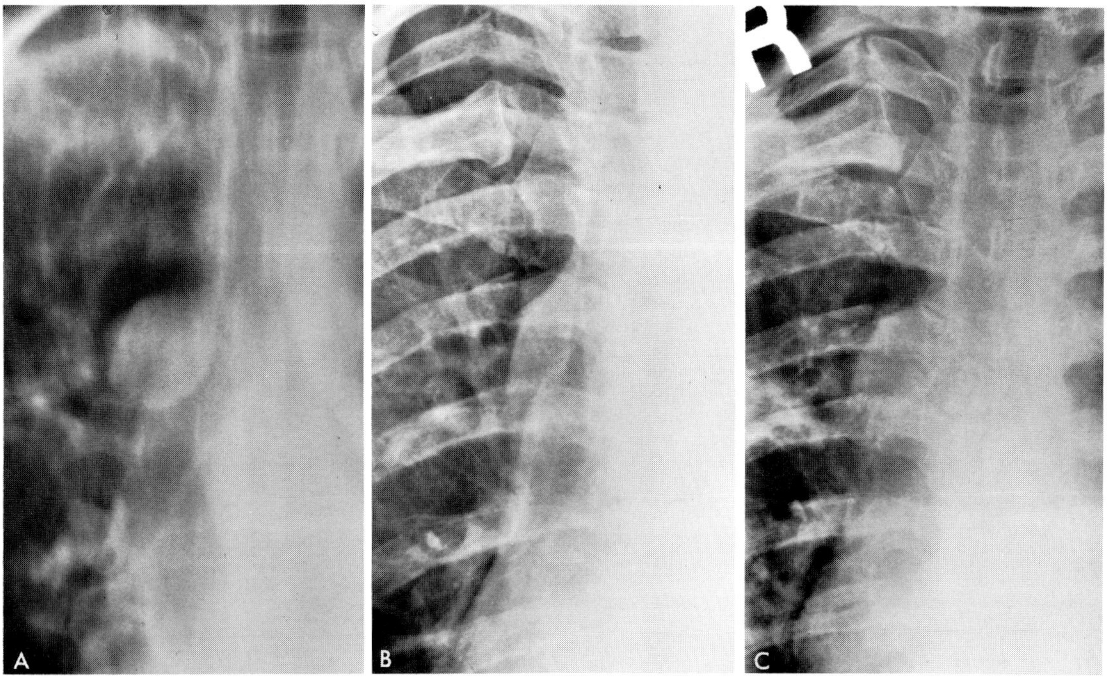

Figure 1–70. **Value of Valsalva and Mueller Procedures in Distinguishing the Vascular or Solid Nature of Intrathoracic Lesions.** *A*, A tomographic section of the mid-mediastinum reveals a well-defined circular shadow situated in the right tracheobronchial angle; differential diagnosis includes an enlarged azygos lymph node or a markedly dilated azygos vein. *B*, A roentgenogram of the same area in the erect position during the Valsalva procedure reveals a marked reduction in the size of the shadow. *C*, A similar projection during the Mueller procedure shows a considerable increase in the size of the shadow compared to *B*. Subsequent angiographic studies proved the shadow to be a markedly dilated azygos vein associated with infradiaphragmatic interruption of the inferior vena cava.

position, a discrepancy which must not be misinterpreted as evidence of disease (Figure 1–69).

Roentgenograms of the chest in many normal erect subjects show more prominent linear markings in the left upper zone than in the corresponding region of the right lung. This asymmetry is understandable in the light of the findings of Dollery and his associates[163] in studies employing lung-scanning techniques with ^{15}oxygen-labeled carbon dioxide; they found significantly greater blood flow through the left than the right upper zone in normal subjects.

Complex interrelationships between transthoracic pressure and pulmonary blood flow occur during inspiration and expiration and during the Valsalva or Mueller maneuver.* It has been established that during inspiration the blood volume increases in the pulmonary arteries and veins and decreases in the capillaries.[164] This change in volume has been documented roentgenographically by Chang,[76] who measured the right descending pulmonary artery in more than 1000 patients and found the caliber consistently larger during inspiration than during expiration in normal subjects, the range of difference being 1 to 3 mm. He found these measurements particularly helpful in the assessment of pulmonary hypertension, in which the inspiratory/expiratory ratio was reversed; this point has been emphasized by Rigler also.[165]

Use of the Valsalva and Mueller maneuvers to produce increase and decrease, respectively, in intra-alveolar pressure has important but limited application in roentgen diagnosis.[166] In 1944 Westermark[167] suggested that increasing the intra-alveolar pressure might prove valuable in differentiating certain diseases of the lungs roentgenographically. He considered that increasing the intra-alveolar pressure reduced the size of congested vessels in pulmonary venous engorgement and "pushed"

*The Valsalva maneuver consists of forced expiration against a closed glottis, and the Mueller maneuver consists of inspiration against a closed glottis. For proper hemodynamic effect, pressures of plus and minus 40 to 50 cm H_2O, respectively, should be maintained for seven to ten seconds. For roentgenograms to be comparable, both maneuvers should be performed at the same degree of lung inflation, preferably at the end of a quiet inspiration.

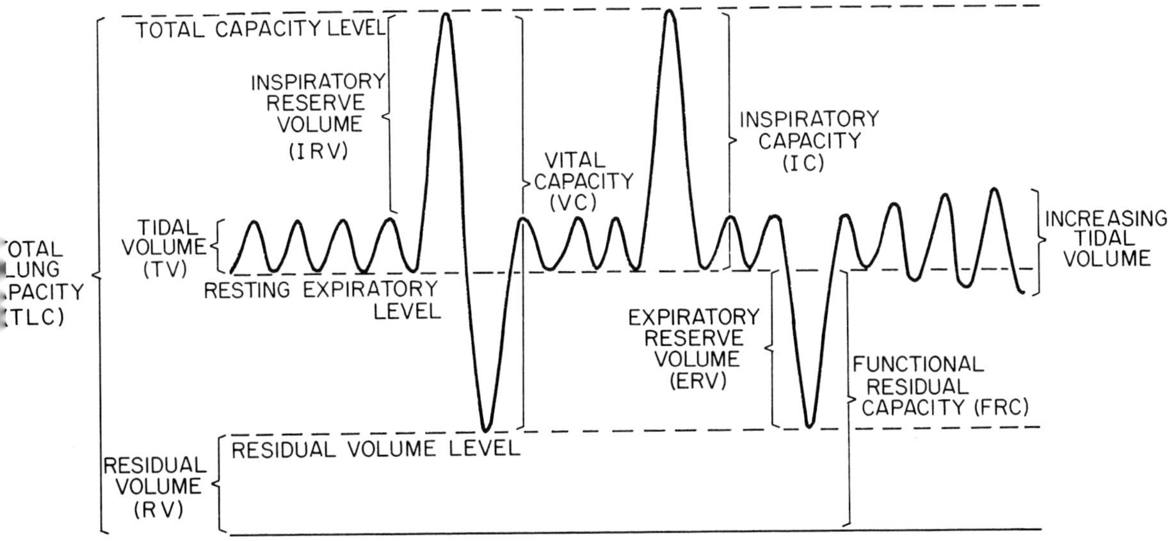

Figure 1–71. **Lung Volumes and Capacities.** *See* text for description.

edema fluid from the airspaces and interstitium back into the vascular tree, thus allowing differentiation of congestion from an infectious process in which this phenomenon did not occur. Although it possesses interesting theoretical possibilities, this technique has proved of little practical value in our experience, partly because congestion and inflammation seldom are confusing entities. However, the Valsalva maneuver may be used to advantage in another context—differentiation of vascular and solid lesions within the thorax:[165, 166] Vascular structures are reduced in size when intra-alveolar pressure is increased, whereas solid lesions remain unchanged. The method is of particular value in the differentiation of an azygos vein from an enlarged azygos lymph node (Figure 1–70), or a pulmonary arteriovenous fistula from a solid mass lesion. Tomography may be employed to considerable advantage during these maneuvers, as pointed out by Amundsen.[168]

These examples of the use of the Valsalva and Mueller maneuvers indicate a trend which has been increasingly emphasized in recent years—the application of physiologic principles to roentgen diagnosis. Knowledge of pathophysiology has played a major role in the roentgenologic study of the cardiovascular system for many years, but it probably has not received the attention in pulmonary diseases that it deserves. A major stimulus to its more frequent application was given by Rigler[165] in 1959, in his classic paper entitled "Functional Roentgen Diagnosis: Anatomical Image—Physiological Interpretation," to which the reader is referred for a concise dissertation on this important topic.

PULMONARY FUNCTION TESTS

Lung Volumes

The volumes and capacities of the lung can be appreciated from a study of the diagram depicted in Figure 1–71. There are four volumes: (1) the tidal volume (TV), which is the amount of gas moving in and out of the lung with each respiratory cycle; (2) the residual volume (RV), which is the amount remaining in the lung after a maximal expiration and is the only lung volume that cannot be measured directly by spirometry; (3) the inspiratory reserve volume (IRV), the additional gas that can be inspired from the end of a quiet inspiration; and (4) the expiratory reserve volume (ERV), the additional amount of gas that can be expired from the resting or end-expiratory level.

There are also four capacities, each of which contains two or more volumes: (a) total lung capacity (TLC), which is the gas contained in the lung at the end of a maximal inspiration; (b) vital capacity (VC), which is the amount that can be expired after a maximal inspiration; (c) inspiratory capacity (IC), which is the amount of gas that can be inspired from the end of a quiet expiration; and (d) functional residual capacity (FRC), which is the volume of gas remaining in the lungs at the end of a quiet expiration.

VITAL CAPACITY (VC) AND ITS SUBDIVISIONS. Although this volume of gas can be measured from the end of a maximal expiration to full inspiration, it is usually expressed as the amount of air expelled from the lungs after a maximal inspiration. In obstructive lung disease, because air is trapped in the lungs, the VC is less when maximal inspiration is followed by maximal expiration than when it is determined from the end of maximal expiration to maximal inspiration. The VC usually is measured with a spirometer; predicted normal values have been calculated based on age, sex, and height.[152] Since there is considerable variation even among normal subjects, no significance should be attached to a measured value that varies 20 per cent or less from the predicted value. The VC also varies depending upon the position of the patient when the volume is recorded; it is less when he is supine than when he is erect.

The VC serves little purpose as an independent measurement of pulmonary function but can be of significant value when considered in conjunction with the results of other tests of pulmonary function. It is a useful index of day-to-day changes in the clinical state of patients with neuromuscular disease. The subdivisions of VC, particularly the inspiratory capacity and inspiratory reserve volume, are rarely useful in assessing pulmonary function. The ERV is greatly reduced in patients with obesity and hypoventilation syndrome, in which state the $\dot{V}A/\dot{Q}$ ratios are low at the lung bases.[111] The TV varies greatly in normal subjects, and the measurement of this by itself usually is not informative; however, multiplication of TV by the respiratory rate per minute yields the minute volume, and in some cases alveolar hypoventilation can be assessed on these two indices alone.

The ratio of measured as a percentage of predicted normal VC to measured as a percentage of predicted normal forced expiratory flow rates (EFR) indicates whether insufficiency is "restrictive" or "obstructive." In obstructive disease the VC is relatively well maintained in comparison with forced EFR, whereas in restrictive disease the EFR may be close to normal and the VC very definitely decreased.

FUNCTIONAL RESIDUAL CAPACITY (FRC) AND RESIDUAL VOLUME (RV). Inert gases are used to measure these compartments. Two methods are commonly used—the open-circuit method, using nitrogen, and the closed-circuit method, using helium. With the open-circuit method the patient breathes 100 per cent oxygen for seven minutes and all expired gas is collected. FRC is calculated by multiplying the amount of gas expired during this period by the percentage of nitrogen in the expired gas. RV is determined by subtracting ERV, as measured on a spirometer, from FRC. With the closed-circuit method the patient breathes from a spirometer containing a known concentration of helium. At the beginning of the experiment the helium concentration in the lungs is zero; as the patient breathes in and out of the spirometer, the gas mixes between spirometer and lungs until the concentration of helium is the same in both. FRC is calculated from the concentration of helium before and at the end of the experiment and the volume in the spirometer. When the lung contains poorly ventilated areas it may be necessary to continue the test for upward of 20 minutes before equilibrium is attained.

The RV is readily obtained by subtracting from FRC the ERV as measured on the spirometer.

When the thorax contains volumes of gas which barely communicate with the conducting tubes, equilibrium between patient and spirometer may appear to be reached while gas is still entering these areas so slowly as to go undetected. To measure the true thoracic gas volume in these circumstances it is necessary to place the patient in a body box (plethysmograph). With this apparatus the thoracic volume can be calculated by applying Boyle's law, which states the relationship between changes in pressure and volume of a gas at constant temperature. The figure obtained, minus FRC determined by the open- or closed-circuit method, is the volume of lung in poor communication with the conducting system.

RV increases with age and in such circumstances does not significantly interfere with function. A marked increase in FRC and RV may occur in the presence of obstructive lung disease; in such cases the volume measured by the body plethysmograph may be higher than that obtained by the open- or closed-circuit method.

In common with VC values, measurements of lung volumes by themselves are of little use in the assessment of lung function, but they may be most informative when considered with the results of other pulmonary function tests.

TOTAL LUNG CAPACITY (TLC). The TLC is calculated simply by the addition of RV and VC. This measurement in itself can be misleading, since TLC may be normal in the presence of serious disease—and, in fact, may be much greater than normal in patients with emphysema, because of increase in the FRC. In "restrictive" disease of the lungs or thoracic cage, the TLC is decreased because of decrease in VC or RV or both.

As with RV and FRC, the TLC may be falsely low when measured by helium and nitrogen methods. Volumetric determination based on posteroanterior and lateral roentgenograms of the chest has been shown to correlate better with values obtained by body plethysmograph in emphysematous patients and may be accomplished by experienced workers in 15 to 20 minutes.[149, 195, 196]

Measurement of Composition of Alveolar Gas

The composition of gas in the acinar unit is dependent upon alveolar ventilation and mixed venous P_{O_2} and P_{CO_2} of the blood in the pulmonary capillaries. The mixed venous blood gases can be determined by analysis of samples obtained through a catheter in the right side of the heart, but this procedure is not suitable for routine use. Mixed venous P_{CO_2} has been measured by a rebreathing method[172, 173] which yields accurate values. The arterial blood P_{CO_2} can be calculated from these results by assuming a constant arterial–venous P_{CO_2} difference of 6 mm.

Ventilation of the acinar unit can be estimated with dependable accuracy in subjects with normal lungs. For this, the total minute ventilation is measured with a spirometer or by collecting expired air in a rubber or plastic bag and determining its volume during passage through a meter. The end-tidal sample accurately reflects the alveolar gas composition in normal lungs; this sample is obtained toward the end of expiration, when the dead space has been washed out. The alveolar ventilation of the normal subject can be calculated from the end-tidal sample of carbon dioxide or oxygen, the volume of expired gas, and the volume and gas content inspired. When the lungs are diseased, however, the situation is not so simple, since there may be many acinar units which are not uniformly ventilated and which empty late in expiration. In such circumstances it is difficult, if not impossible, to obtain a true alveolar (or acinar) sample, and a reliable estimate of alveolar ventilation requires measurement of the total minute ventilation and subtraction from this of an assumed volume of anatomic dead space, based on several factors, including age, sex, FRC, and tidal volume. The volume of alveolar ventilation per minute of a patient with diseased lungs may equal that of a subject with healthy lungs of the same age, sex, and build. Despite the fact that the patient has some units which are barely ventilated, he has others that are overventilated, and, therefore, total ventilation may be normal.

There is no doubt, however, that the most accurate index of alveolar ventilation is analysis of an arterial blood sample, which gives values for P_{CO_2} and P_{O_2}. This is considered in greater detail later, but it can be said here that a P_{CO_2} value above the normal range indicates that many acinar units are poorly ventilated.

Measurement of Mechanics of Acinar Ventilation

MEASUREMENT OF COMPLIANCE. Compliance is the relationship between the pressure required to overcome "elastic recoil" and the volume of air that moves into the lung as a result of this pressure change. To avoid the effect of resistance, and to measure compliance alone, the test is done in a "static" position, that is, while the breath is held with the glottis open. As the normal lung becomes more inflated it becomes less compliant and the pressure-volume curve becomes more horizontal (*see* Figure 1–72). Compliance is expressed in liters/cm H_2O. Pressure is measured by a manometer attached to a tube leading to a thin-walled balloon which is swallowed to the mid-esophagus. The volume is measured either by use of a pneumotachograph at the mouth, with integration of the pneumotachogram signal, or while the patient breathes from a spirometer. This pressure-volume curve includes measurement of the "elastic" properties of the elastic and collagen tissues of the lungs and those of the thoracic cage and the force required to overcome the surface-tension effect of the alveoli. The surface-ac-

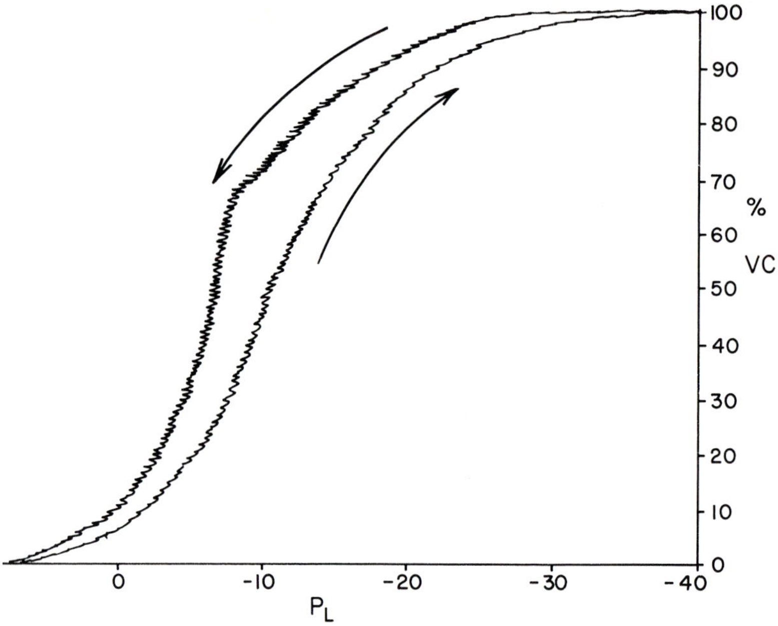

Figure 1–72. **Pressure–volume Curve.** A pressure–volume tracing of a young male adult measured in both inspiration and expiration from residual volume to total lung capacity and back to residual volume. The upper curve represents the expiratory tracing. Notice the more horizontal appearance (decrease in compliance) as total lung capacity is reached.

tive properties of removed lung tissue can be measured, but no technique has been devised to determine the surface-lining tension *in vivo.*

MEASUREMENT OF RESISTANCE

Spirometry. These are indirect methods for determining the resistance of the airways and lung tissue. A single forced inspiratory or expiratory curve is measured on a revolving drum or a bellows-type apparatus and is expressed as liters/sec moved in or out of the lung. In patients with obstructive lung disease a simple spirogram during deep breathing often shows the longer expiration than inspiration and the air-trapping that occurs after maximal inspiration. The "timed vital capacity" may be used to quantify expiration; after an inspiration, the patient exhales as rapidly as he can all of the air in his lungs. This is the forced expiratory volume (FEV); the amount expired during the first 0.75 second, the first 1.0 second, and the first 3.0 seconds, are expressed $FEV_{0.75}$, $FEV_{1.0}$, and $FEV_{3.0}$. Normal persons exhale approximately 83 per cent of VC in 1.0 second and approximately 97 per cent in 3.0 seconds, whereas expiratory flow curves of patients with obstructive lung disease are prolonged. On the other hand, although patients with a restrictive lung condition such as fibrosis may have a substantially reduced VC, they can have almost normal $FEV_{1.0}$ and $FEV_{3.0}$ values, since there is no bronchial obstruction.

Many ways of expressing the forced-expiration curve have been devised. In our laboratory we measure FEV on a rapidly revolving drum and from this curve determine $FEV_{0.75}$ (the volume expired in the first three-quarters of a second), which is multiplied by 40 and is expressed in liters/min. This is sometimes referred to as the indirect maximal breathing capacity (MBC) or maximal voluntary ventilation (MVV) (*see the following discussion*), since it has been shown that, in normal subjects, $FEV_{0.75} \times 40$ closely correlates with direct measurement of the MBC or MVV. In addition, we measure the middle half of the FEV curve and express this volume in liters/sec (Figure 1–73).

In place of the single forced expiratory curve recorded on a spirometer, measurement of the maximal volume of gas that can be breathed per minute is used in some laboratories; this also is known as the MBC or MVV. It can be calculated from a tracing made while the patient breathes in and out of a spirometer as rapidly as possible for 15 seconds, or by collecting the expired gas in a bag for the same length of time. The value is multiplied by four to give the volume in liters/min. Since this test is very tiring, particularly for patients with abnormal lungs, it is used less and less.

Although these indirect methods for assessing resistance in the lungs are simple to perform and are widely used, they must be

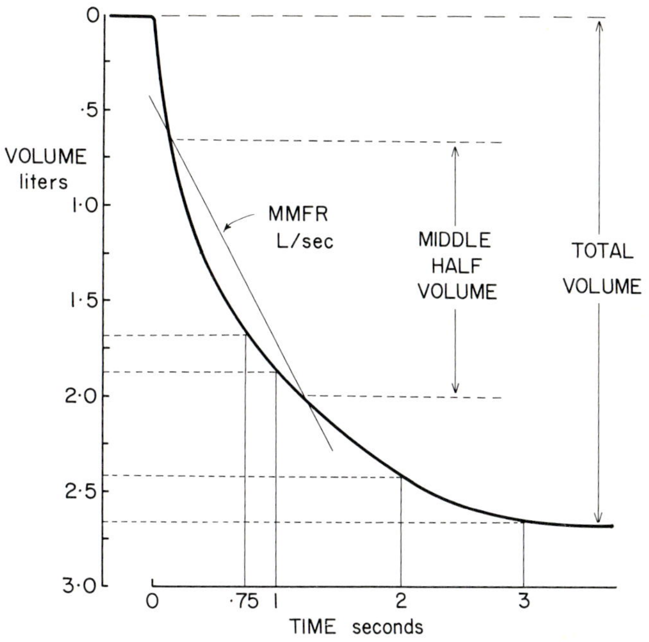

Figure 1–73. **Measurement of Ventilatory Volumes.** This graph depicts the curve of a forced vital capacity (FVC) in which a total volume of 2.6 liters has been expired in 3 seconds ($FEV_{3.0}$). Volumes expired during the 3/4 second ($FEV_{0.75}$), 1 second ($FEV_{1.0}$), and 2 second ($FEV_{2.0}$) intervals are also indicated. The maximal midexpiratory flow rate (MMFR) can be calculated at 1.3 liters/sec.

interpreted with caution: (1) the test requires the co-operation of the patient, and falsely low values may be recorded and (2) it does not indicate specific mechanical abnormalities, since patients with decreased compliance have reduced flow rates, and, therefore, direct measurements of resistance are preferable.

Use of Body Plethysmograph. Since resistance equals the pressure difference divided by the volume flow, resistance in the airways can be determined only with knowledge of the instantaneous air flow and the difference between atmospheric and alveolar pressures. Air flow can be determined with a pneumotachograph, but the measurement of alveolar pressure requires a more elaborate procedure. The patient breathes in and out in an airtight box and the pressure around him is measured and recorded by a very sensitive manometer. The alveolar pressure can be calculated from the change in pressure in the box during the respiratory cycle.

Use of Mouth Pressure For Determining Airway Resistance. Alveolar pressure can be determined indirectly by using an electrically controlled shutter; while this device momentarily shuts off flow during inspiration, the mouth pressure (which, presumably, is equal to the alveolar pressure immediately before interruption) is recorded. The apparatus is cheaper but yields less accurate values than the body plethysmograph.

Normal values as determined by the body plethysmograph during rapid, shallow breathing range from 0.6 to 2.4 cm H_2O/liter/sec, with flow rates of 0.5 liter/sec in adults.

Measurement of Perfusion of Acinar Units

MEASUREMENT OF VOLUME, FLOW, AND PRESSURE. Although volume, pressure, and flow of blood in individual acinar units cannot be determined, their values in the lungs as a whole can be measured during catheterization of the right side of the heart. Cardiac output can be measured while the patient is resting or exercising, using the Fick method or dye-dilution curves. Instantaneous pulmonary capillary flow (V_C) can be measured by two methods. In the first, the patient inhales a mixture of 80 per cent nitrous oxide and 20 per cent oxygen while seated in a body plethysmograph; the sensitive manometer which records the pressure around the patient shows an abrupt fall as nitrous oxide leaves the acini to dissolve in the blood. Carbon monoxide is used in the second method to measure diffusion; the membrane component can be separated from that due to the blood, and V_C can be estimated.[77, 78]

MEASUREMENT OF THE DISTRIBUTION OF CAPILLARY BLOOD. The relative V_C to each lung can be determined from the oxygen uptake recorded during bronchospirometry, in which a special catheter is introduced through the trachea, separating the conducting system to each lung. The oxygen uptake of individual lobes can be measured, but this technique is not suitable for routine use in even the most sophisticated laboratories. Newer methods for determining the distribution of pulmonary capillary blood make use of a radioactive gas, such as xenon; this is injected and its regional distribution throughout the lungs is measured by scintillation counters placed over the chest wall. Radioactive carbon dioxide, which is inhaled, can be used similarly. These methods are still gross and do not detect the distribution of blood to the barely macroscopic acinar unit. Further reference is made to this technique in the discussion of ventilation/perfusion ratios.

Measurement of the Diffusion of Gas in Acinar Units

The diffusing capacity formerly was calculated directly from the diffusion of oxygen; carbon monoxide has largely replaced this gas, for technical reasons. The diffusing capacity for carbon monoxide (DL_{CO}) is computed as follows:

$$DL_{co} = \frac{\text{ml of CO taken up by capillary blood}}{\text{mean alveolar PCO} - \text{mean capillary PCO.}}$$

The amount of carbon monoxide taken up by capillary blood is calculated by subtracting volume × CO concentration of expired gas from volume × CO concentration of inspired gas. Determination of the denominator of this equation is more subject to error in cases of lung diseases. In normal subjects, a sample of gas expired at the end of tidal volume reflects accurately the mean alveolar P_{CO}, and, since the normal mean capillary P_{CO} is so small that it can be ignored, the diffusing capacity can be calculated reliably. However, in diseased lungs which have relatively underventilated areas that empty late, the normal sharp division between dead-space gas and alveolar gas is lost and the end-tidal sample does not necessarily represent the mean alveolar P_{CO}.

Several techniques for use with carbon monoxide have been devised for measuring the diffusing capacity. The main differences between these techniques are the length of time the carbon monoxide is kept in the lungs and the methods of determining the mean alveolar P_{CO}. The single-breath method entails the inhalation of a gas which contains minute quantities of carbon monoxide and breath-holding for ten seconds. The steady-state technique requires the inhalation of the carbon monoxide gas mixture for several breaths, until alveolar P_{CO} remains constant. We use the steady-state method and determine mean alveolar P_{CO} from an end-tidal sample under resting conditions. In addition to the diffusing capacity, the fractional removal of carbon monoxide is calculated from the end-tidal sample; this confirms the accuracy of the diffusing-capacity value, since both decrease simultaneously in the majority of cases.[174]

The fractional uptake of carbon monoxide is the amount removed divided by the amount inspired; thus:

$$\text{CO uptake (\%)} = \frac{\text{CO inspired} - \text{CO expired}}{\text{CO inspired}}.$$

During hyperventilation, fractional carbon monoxide uptake may decrease but the diffusing capacity is unchanged. During hypoventilation, however, the diffusing capacity may be reduced due to a very low tidal volume, whereas fractional carbon monoxide uptake decreases to a lesser extent. Diffusing capacity during exercise can be determined by the steady-state method; however, an end-tidal sample obtained in these circumstances is not reliable, and since the numerator of the equation for calculating the diffusing capacity for carbon monoxide becomes the chief determinant, in such instances it is valid to calculate alveolar P_{CO} from the inspired and expired carbon monoxide concentrations, assuming a value for the respiratory dead space.

The diffusing capacity reflects not only the thickness of the alveolocapillary membrane but also the total area of this membrane and the hemoglobin content of the pulmonary capillary blood. Removal of a lobe or an entire lung reduces the overall diffusing area. Inequality in the ventilation/perfusion ratio results in a decrease in the diffusing capacity, because less carbon monoxide is taken up by poorly ventilated or poorly perfused areas than by areas with normal perfusion and ventilation. Since the uptake of carbon monoxide by capillary blood is due mainly to its great affinity for hemoglobin, in cases of anemia the diffusing capacity may be reduced because of hemoglobin lack. During exercise, the increased size of the pulmonary vascular bed and increased cardiac output cause increase in the diffusing capacity.

Measurement of Matching of Blood Flow and Ventilation

MEASUREMENTS OF DISTRIBUTION OF INSPIRED AIR. Poorly ventilated acinar units receive less oxygen from a single deep breath of 100 per cent oxygen and empty later during the next expiration than well-ventilated acini. This is the rationale of the single-breath 100 per cent oxygen test with continuous analysis by nitrogen meter of the expired air. After a single inspiration of 100 per cent oxygen, the first part of the expiration contains 100 per cent oxygen, which comes from the dead space. Next, the expired gas comes from the acini; if these empty synchronously and are equally ventilated the nitrogen meter curve shows a horizontal line throughout the rest of the expiration. Poorly ventilated acini receive smaller amounts of oxygen and empty late so that during the next complete expiration the nitrogen curve slopes upward as it records their contribution.

The percentage of nitrogen expired can be calculated in a multiple-breath method during which the patient breathes 100 per cent oxygen for seven minutes. When the distribution of inspired air is uniform the nitrogen content of an "alveolar" sample at the end of the seven minutes is 2.5 per cent or less. In patients with impaired distribution, 10 to 20 minutes may elapse before the nitrogen content of poorly ventilated areas has been replaced by oxygen, and the nitrogen content of an "alveolar" sample taken at the end of seven minutes may greatly exceed the normal figure of 2.5 per cent.

The third method for determining the distribution of inspired gas makes use of the helium closed-circuit apparatus and is expressed as the mixing efficiency (ME). This apparatus can be used to calculate lung volumes also, including RV. The patient is connected to the circuit and breathes from a spirometer containing helium,[174] and the concentration of expired gas is measured by a katharometer; the distribution is determined by recording the number of breaths taken before the helium concentration remains steady.

MEASUREMENT OF DISTRIBUTION OF PULMONARY CAPILLARY BLOOD. Uneven distribution of pulmonary capillary blood in the presence of relatively uniform ventilation can be detected when the areas of unperfused lung are large. The alveolar P_{CO_2} is determined by analysis of a sample of expired gas taken at the end of tidal volume (end-tidal) or at the end of maximal expiration (end-expiratory) and is compared with the arterial P_{CO_2}. A P_{CO_2} difference of greater than 6 mm Hg indicates the presence of large numbers of unperfused acini; the expired gas from these areas contains no carbon dioxide and, therefore, decreases the P_{CO_2} of the total sample of gas. This measurement becomes less accurate with the development of compensatory mechanisms which decrease ventilation to unperfused areas and divert inspired air to those that are well perfused.

MEASUREMENT OF INEQUALITY OF VENTILATION/PERFUSION RATIOS. Unlike the single-breath method, which utilizes an inert gas that measures the distribution of inspired air only, continuous analysis of a single expiration by means of a carbon dioxide analyzer gives information pertaining to both ventilation and perfusion and their uniformity. A rise in the carbon dioxide concentration throughout expiration indicates perfusion of poorly ventilated areas which empty late in the expiratory phase.

An increase in the "physiologic" dead space, which can be calculated with the Bohr equation,[1] is another method for assessing inequality of ventilation/perfusion. Inequality when there is overperfusion relative to ventilation is manifested by an increase in the alveolar-arterial difference for nitrogen (A–a N_2). In poorly ventilated areas which are perfused the P_{O_2} is decreased, whereas the P_{CO_2} and P_{N_2} are increased. The arterial blood P_{N_2} is reflected in the P_{N_2} of the urine, and the A–a N_2 can be determined by gas chromatography without the necessity for arterial puncture. Since nitrogen is an inert gas, the venous blood and arterial blood P_{N_2} are identical. Thus, a true or "absolute" shunt of venous to arterial blood effects no change in the alveolo-arterial nitrogen difference, and, since there appears to be no alveolar-end-capillary difference for nitrogen, this test can be used to rule out blood-shunt and diffusion defect to confirm whether hypoxemia is due to ventilation/perfusion inequality. In other words, a difference in nitrogen values in arterial blood (or urine) and alveolar gas can result only from inequality of ventilation/perfusion ratios, due to the perfusion of poorly ventilated areas.

Bronchospirometry is used to detect differences in ventilation and perfusion in the two lungs. When oxygen uptake is decreased and ventilation to one lung is normal or nearly so, perfusion is abnormal.

In recent years, tests have been devised which not only detect the presence of ventilation/perfusion inequality in the lung but also its location. These methods are still in their infancy and necessitate expensive equipment, but results obtained so far are so spectacular that undoubtedly these techniques will be widely used in routine pulmonary function assessment in the future. This use of radioactive oxygen and carbon dioxide was summarized in a recent monograph by West,[107] and the inhalation and intravenous injection of radioactive xenon to show the distribution of inspired gas and the perfusion of pulmonary capillaries has been used by workers in the Cardio-respiratory Service of the Royal Victoria Hospital.[102, 190–194]

Measurement of Blood Gases and H^+ ion Concentration

Arterial blood can be obtained almost as easily as venous blood. Brachial or radial arteries should be used in preference to femoral arteries, which should be punctured only as a last resort. Since arteries are deeper than veins they are more evasive; therefore, the area should be infiltrated with local anesthetic, which serves the double purpose of reducing pain and vasospasm. It is no longer necessary to use a Cournand or Riley needle for routine arterial puncture; we use very sharp disposable needles which fit tightly on to the adapter of a 10 or 20 ml syringe. A heparin solution is drawn through the needle and allowed to coat the sides of the syringe, and then all of the air and heparin is expelled. The needle is introduced at an angle of 45 to 90 degrees at the site of maximal pulsation; a pulsatile flow into the syringe is seen when the lumen of the vessel is entered. It is wise to maintain pressure on the site of puncture for five to ten minutes after withdrawal of the needle. The orifice of the needle is immediately sealed with a rubber stopper; any air which gets into the barrel of the syringe should be expelled before the needle is stopped. Results are most accurate when the sample is analyzed immediately; when this is not possible the sample should be placed in a refrigerator.

The Van Slyke method of measuring oxygen content and oxygen capacity of arterial blood is used still in the modern pulmonary function laboratory as a yardstick for checking the accuracy of newer methods. In our routine laboratory we use a spectrophotometric method (Beckman Instruments, Inc., Fullerton, California) to determine the arterial oxygen saturation, and we simultaneously measure the P_{O_2} of the arterial blood with an electrode (Instrument Laboratories, Inc., Watertown, Mass.). This assessment of arterial blood oxygen by two methods is useful for detecting technical errors, since the accuracy of values can be ascertained by reference to the oxygen dissociation curve.

P_{CO_2} and H^+ ion concentration also can be measured with electrodes (Instrument Laboratories, Inc., Watertown, Mass.). It is essential that the accuracy of these delicate instruments be checked from time to time, using an Astrup apparatus to make duplicate measurements.

In infants or young children arterialized capillary blood samples may be obtained from the finger or heel with a heparinized capillary tube and the results compare favorably with simultaneously obtained arterial blood.[197]

REFERENCES

1. Bates, David V., and Christie, R. V.: Respiratory Function in Disease. Philadelphia, W. B. Saunders, 1964.
2. Comroe, Julius H., Jr.: Pulmonary arterial blood flow: effects of brief and permanent arrest. Amer. Rev. Resp. Dis., *85*:179-190, 1962.
3. Comroe, J. H., Jr.: Physiology of Respiration. Chicago, Year Book Medical Publishers, 1965.
4. Miller, William S.: The Lung. Springfield, Ill., Charles C Thomas, 1937.
5. Aschoff, L.: Lectures on Pathology. New York, Hoeber, 1924, pp. 53-57.
6. Weill, Hans, Ferrans, V. J., Gay, R. M., and Ziskind, M. M.: Early lipoid pneumonia: roentgenologic, anatomic and physiologic characteristics. Amer. J. Med., *36*:370-376, 1964.
7. Loeshcke, H.: Die Morphologie des normalen und emphysemetösen Acinus der Lunge. Beitr. Z. Path. Anat., *68*:213-223, 1921.
8. Pump, K. K.: The morphology of the finer branches of the bronchial tree of the human lung. Dis. Chest, *46*:379-398, 1964.
9. Weibel, Ewald R.: Morphometry of the Human Lung. New York, Academic Press Inc., 1963.
10. Tyler, W. S., and Pearse, A. G. E.: Oxidative enzymes of the interalveolar septum of the rat. Thorax, *20*:149-152, 1965.
11. Azzopardi, A., and Thurlbeck, W. M.: The oxidative enzyme pattern in developing and adult mice and adult rabbits. Lab Invest., *16*:706-716, 1967.
12. Thurlbeck, William M.: The internal surface area of nonemphysematous lungs. Amer. Rev. Resp. Dis., *95*:765-773, 1967.
13. Schultze, G.: Unusual roentgen manifestations of primary staphylococcal pneumonia in infants and young children. Amer. J. Roentgen., *81*:290-295, 1959.
14. Lambert, Margaret Waugh: Accessory bronchiole-alveolar communications. J. Path. Bact., *70*:311-314, 1955.
15. von Hayek, Heinrich: The Human Lung. New York, Hafner, 1960.
16. Martin, H. B.: Respiratory bronchioles as the pathway for collateral ventilation. J. Appl. Physiol., *21*:1443-1447, 1966.
17. Sherrick, D. W., Kincaid, O. W., and DuShane, J. W.: Agenesis of a main branch of the pulmonary artery. Amer. J. Roentgen., *87*:917-928, 1962.
18. Twining, E. W.: In Shanks, S. C., and Kerley, P. (eds.), A Textbook of X-ray Diagnosis, Vol. II (2nd ed.). Philadelphia, W. B. Saunders, 1951, 1951, pp. 208–209.
19. Ziskind, Morton M., Weill, H., and Payzant, A. R.: The recognition and significance of acinus-filling processes of the lungs. Amer. Rev. Resp. Dis., *87*:551-559, 1963.
20. Ziskind, M. M., Weill, H., Buechner, H. A., and Brown, M.: Recognition of distinctive radiologic patterns in diffuse pulmonary disease. Arch. Intern. Med., *114*:108-112, 1964.
21. Felson, B.: The roentgen diagnosis of disseminated pulmonary alveolar diseases. Seminars in Roentgen., *2*:3-21, 1967.
22. Staub, Norman C.: The interdependence of pulmonary structure and function. Anesthesiol., *24*:831-854, 1963.
23. Pump, K. K.: The circulation in the peripheral parts of the human lung. Dis. Chest, *49*:119-129, 1966.
24. von Hayek, H.: Cellular structure and mucus activity in the bronchial tree and alveoli. In: deReuck, A. V. S., and O'Connor, M. (eds.), Ciba Foundation: Symposium on Pulmonary Structure and Function. London, J. & A. Churchill, 1962, p. 100.
25. Clara, Max: Zur Histobiologie des Bronchalepithels. Z. mikr.-anat. Forsch., *41*:321-347, 1937.
26. de Haller, R., and Reid, L.: Adult chronic bronchitis. Morphology, histochemistry and vascularization of the bronchial mucous glands. Med. Thorac., *22*:549-567, 1965.
27. Boyden, Edward A., and Hartmann, J. Francis: An analysis of variations in the bronchopulmonary segments of the left upper lobes of fifty lungs. Amer. J. Anat., *79*:321-360, 1946.
28. Boyden, Edward A., and Scannell, J. Gordon: An analysis of variations in the bronchovascular pattern of the right upper lobe of fifty lungs. Amer. J. Anat., *82*:27-72, 1948.
29. Scannell, J. Gordon: A study of variations of the bronchopulmonary segments in the left upper lobe. J. Thoracic Surg., *16*:530-537, 1947.
30. Scannell, J. Gordon, and Boyden, E. A.: A study of variations of the bronchopulmonary segments of the right upper lobe. J. Thoracic Surg., *17*:232-237, 1948.
31. Scannell, J. Gordon: An anatomic approach to segmental resection. J. Thorac. Surg., *18*:64-74, 1949.
32. Smith, Franklin R., and Boyden, E. A.: An analysis of variations of the segmental bronchi of the right lower lobe of fifty injected lungs. J. Thorac. Surg., *18*:195-215, 1949.
33. Boyden, E. A., and Hamre, C. J.: An analysis of

variations in the bronchovascular patterns of the middle lobe in fifty dissected and twenty injected lungs. J. Thorac. Surg., *21*:172-188, 1951.
34. Boyden, Edward A.: Segmental Anatomy of the Lungs. New York, McGraw Hill, 1955.
35. Bloomer, W. E., Liebow, A. A., and Hales, M. R.: Surgical Anatomy of the Bronchovascular Segments. Springfield, Ill., Charles C Thomas, 1960.
36. Jackson, Chevalier L., and Huber, John Franklin: Correlated applied anatomy of the bronchial tree and lungs with system of nomenclature. Dis. Chest, *9*:319-326, 1943.
37. Brock, R. C. (member of the Sub-Committee): The nomenclature of broncho-pulmonary anatomy. An international nomenclature accepted by the Thoracic Society. Thorax, *5*:222-228, 1950.
38. Fraser, Robert G.: Measurements of the calibre of human bronchi in three phases of respiration by cinebronchography. J. Canad. Ass. Radiol., *12*:102-112, 1961.
39. Merendino, K. Alvin, and Kiriluk, Lawrence B.: Human measurements involved in tracheobronchial resection and reconstruction procedures; report of case of bronchial adenoma. Surgery, *35*:590-597, 1954.
40. Jesseph, John E., and Merendino, K. Alvin: The dimensional interrelationships of the major components of the human tracheobronchial tree. Surg. Gynec. Obstet., *105*:210-214, 1957.
41. Nelson, S.: Personal communication, 1965.
42. Pierce, John A., and Ebert, R. V.: Fibrous network of the lung and its change with age. Thorax, *20*:469-476, 1965.
43. Oderr, Charles: Architecture of the lung parenchyma: studies with a specially designed x-ray microscope. Amer. Rev. Resp. Dis., *90*:401-410, 1964.
44. von Neegaard, K.: Neue Auffassungen über einen Grundbegriff der Atemmechanik: Die Retraktionskraft der Lunge, abhängig von der Oberflächenspannung in den Alveolen. Z. Ges. Exp. Med., *66*:373-394, 1929.
45. Pattle, R. E.: Properties, function and origin of the alveolar lining layer. Nature, *175*:1125-1126, 1955.
46. Pattle, R. E.: A test of silicone anti-foam treatment of lung oedema in rabbits. J. Path. Bact., *72*:203-209, 1956.
47. Radford, Edward P., Jr.: Method for estimating respiratory surface area of mammalian lungs from their physical characteristics. Proc. Soc. Exp. Biol. Med., *87*:58-61, 1954.
48. Clements, J. A.: Dependence of pressure-volume characteristics of lungs on intrinsic surface-active material. Amer. J. Physiol., *187*:592, (abstr.) 1956.
49. Clements, John A.: Surface tension of lung extracts. Proc. Soc. Exp. Biol. Med., *95*:170-172, 1957.
50. Tierney, Donald F.: Pulmonary surfactant in health and disease. Dis. Chest, *47*:247-253, 1965.
51. Mead, Jere, and Collier, C.: Relation of volume history of lungs to respiratory mechanics in anesthetized dogs. J. Appl. Physiol., *14*:669-678, 1959.
52. Klaus, M., Reiss, O. K., Tooley, W. H., Piel, C., and Clements, J. A.: Alveolar epithelial cell mitochondria as source of the surface-active lung lining. Science, *137*:750-751, 1962.
53. Avery, Mary Ellen, and Mead, Jere: Surface properties in relation to atelectasis and hyaline membrane disease. A.M.A.J. Dis. Child., *97*:517-523, 1959.
54. Tooley, W. H., Finley, T. N., and Gardner, R.: Some effects on the lungs of blood from a pump oxygenator. (Abstract, American Physiological Society Proceedings, Fall Meeting, Sept. 5-8, 1961) Physiologist, *4*:124, 1961 (August).
55. Pattle, R. E.: The lining layer of the lung alveoli. Brit. Med. Bull., *19*:41-44, 1963.
56. Mead, Jere: Mechanical properties of lungs. Physiol. Rev., *41*:281-330, 1961.
57. Clements, John A.: Surfactant in pulmonary disease. New Eng. J. Med., *272*:1336-1337, 1965.
58. Dayman, Howard: Mechanics of airflow in health and in emphysema. J. Clin. Invest., *30*:1175-1190, 1951.
59. DiRienzo, S.: Bronchial dynamism. Radiology, *53*:168-186, 1949.
60. Wright, Robert R.: Bronchial atrophy and collapse in chronic obstructive pulmonary emphysema. Amer. J. Path., *37*:63-77, 1960.
61. Macklem, Peter T., Fraser, R. G., and Bates, D. V.: Bronchial pressures and dimensions in health and obstructive airway disease. J. Appl. Physiol., *18*:699-706, 1963.
62. Macklem, P. T.: Personal communication, 1968.
63. Colebatch, H. J. H., Olsen, C. R., and Nadel, J. A.: Effects of intravenous histamine and 48/80 on lung mechanics. Fed. Proc. *21*/(Abstr. 337), 445, 1962.
64. Swenson, E. W., Finley, T. N., and Guzman, S. V.: Unilateral hypoventilation in man during temporary occlusion of one pulmonary artery. J. Clin. Invest., *40*:828-835, 1961.
65. Severinghaus, John W., Swenson, E. W., Finley, T. N., Lategola, M. T., and Williams, J.: Unilateral hypoventilation produced in dogs by occluding one pulmonary artery. J. Appl. Physiol., *16*:53-60, 1961.
66. Elliott, F. M., and Reid, L.: Some new facts about the pulmonary artery and its branching pattern. Clin. Radiol., *16*:193-198, 1965.
67. Liebow, A.: Recent advances in pulmonary anatomy. In: de Reuck, A. V. S., and O'Connor, M. (eds.), Ciba Foundation: Symposium on Pulmonary Structure and Function. London, J. & A. Churchill, 1962, pp. 17-19.
68. Turner-Warwick, Margaret: Systemic arterial patterns in the lung and clubbing of the fingers. Thorax, *18*:238-250, 1963.
69. Felson, B.: Fundamentals of Chest Roentgenology. Philadelphia, W. B. Saunders, 1960.
70. Jefferson, K. E.: The normal pulmonary angiogram and some changes seen in chronic nonspecific lung disease. I. The pulmonary vessels in the normal pulmonary angiogram. Proc. Roy. Soc. Med., *58*:677-681, 1965.
71. Hornykiewytsch, T. H., and Stender, H. St.: Normale und pathologisch veränderte Lungengefässe in Schichtbild. Fortschr. Roentgenstr., *79*:44-51, 1953.
72. Fraser, R. G., and Bates, D. V.: Body section roentgenography in the evaluation and differentiation of chronic hypertrophic emphysema and asthma. Amer. J. Roentgen., *82*:39-62, 1959.

73. Michelson, Elliot, and Salik, J. O.: The vascular pattern of the lung as seen on routine and tomographic studies. Radiology, *73*:511-526, 1959.
74. Wójtowicz, Jerzy: Some tomographic criteria for an evaluation of the pulmonary circulation. Acta Radiol. (Diagn.), *2*:215-224, 1964.
75. Simon, G.: The lateral position in chest tomography. J. Fac. Radiol., *4*:77-88, 1952.
76. Chang, C. H. (Joseph): The normal roentgenographic measurement of the right descending pulmonary artery in 1,085 cases. Amer. J. Roentgen., *87*:929-935, 1962.
77. Roughton, F. J. W., and Forster, R. E.: Relative importance of diffusion and chemical reaction rates in determining rate of exchange of gases in the human lung, with special reference to true diffusing capacity of pulmonary membrane and volume of blood in the lung capillaries. J. Appl. Physiol., *11*:290-302, 1957.
78. Bates, D. V., Varvis, C. J., Donevan, R. E., and Christie, R. V.: Variations in the pulmonary capillary blood volume and membrane diffusion component in health and disease. J. Clin. Invest., *39*:1401-1412, 1960.
79. Newman, Faith, Smalley, B. F., and Thomson, M. L.: Effect of exercise, body and lung size on CO diffusion in athletes and nonathletes. J. Appl. Physiol., *17*:649-655, 1962.
80. Johnson, Robert L., Jr., Taylor, H. F., and Lawson, W. H., Jr., with the technical assistance of Prengler: Maximal diffusing capacity of the lung for carbon monoxide. J. Clin. Invest., *44*:349-355, 1965.
81. Weibel, Ewald R.: Morphometrische Analyse von Zahl, Volumen und Oberfläche der Alveolen und Kapillären der menschlichen Lunge. Z. Zell-Forsch., *57*:648-666, 1962.
82. Cander, Leon, and Forster, R. E.: Determination of pulmonary parenchymal tissue volume and pulmonary capillary blood flow in man. J. Appl. Physiol., *14*:541-551, 1959.
83. Caro, C. G.: Physics of blood flow in the lung. Brit. Med. Bull., *19*:66-70, 1963.
84. Altmann, Kurt: Experimentell-morphologische Untersuchungen über die Beziehungen zwischen der Lungencapillärweite und dem Lungendehnurgsgrad. Z. Ges. Exp. Med., *122*:516-548, 1954.
85. Permutt, Solbert, Howell, J. B. L., Proctor, D. F., and Riley, R. L.: Effect of lung inflation on static pressure-volume characteristics of pulmonary vessels. J. Appl. Physiol., *16*:64-70, 1961.
86. Olkon, D. M., and Joannides, M.: The capillary circulation in the alveolus pulmonalis of the living dog. Arch. Intern. Med., *45*:201-205, 1930.
87. Ramos, J. Garcia: On the dynamics of the lung's capillary circulation. I. The mechanical factors. Amer. Rev. Tuberc., *71*:822-829, 1955.
88. Dubois, Arthur B., and Marshall, R.: Measurements of pulmonary capillary blood flow and gas exchange throughout the respiratory cycle in man. J. Clin. Invest., *36*:1566-1571, 1957.
89. Staub, Norman C., and Storey, W. F.: Relation between morphological and physiological events in lung studied by rapid freezing. J. Appl. Physiol., *17*:381-390, 1962.
90. Simmons, Daniel H., Linde, Leonard M., and Shapiro, Bertrand J.: Effect of blood gases and acid-base disturbances on the pulmonary circulation. Dis. Chest, *48*:347-350, 1965.
91. Fishman, Alfred P.: Respiratory gases in the regulation of the pulmonary circulation. Physiol. Rev., *41*:214-280, 1961.
92. Staub, Norman C.: Site of action of hypoxia on the pulmonary vasculature. Fed. Proc. *22*: (Abstr. 1748), 453, 1963.
93. Dexter, L., Dow, J. W., Haynes, F. W., Whittenberger, J. L., Ferris, B. G., Goodale, W. T., and Hellems, H. K.: Studies of the pulmonary circulation in man at rest. Normal variations and the interrelations between increased pulmonary blood flow, elevated pulmonary arterial pressure, and high pulmonary "capillary" pressures. J. Clin. Invest., *29*:602-613, 1950.
94. Gorlin, R., Haynes, F. W., Goodale, W. T., Sawyer, C. G., Dow, J. W., and Dexter, L.: Studies of circulatory dynamics in mitral stenosis. II. Altered dynamics at rest. Amer. Heart J., *41*:30-45, 1951.
95. Cudkowicz, L., and Wraith, D. G.: A method of study of the pulmonary circulation in finger clubbing. Thorax, *12*:313-320, 1957.
96. Liebow, Averill A.: Recent observations on pulmonary collateral circulation. Med. Thorac., *19*:609-622, 1962.
97. Schulz, H.: Die submikroskopische Anatomie und Pathologie der Lunge. (The submicroscopic anatomy and pathology of the lung.) Berlin, Springer, 1959.
98. Finley, T. N., Swenson, E. W., and Comroe, J. H., Jr.: The cause of arterial hypoxemia at rest in patients with "alveolar-capillary block syndrome." J. Clin. Invest., *41*:618-622, 1962.
99. Read, John, and Williams, R. S.: Pulmonary ventilation: blood flow relationships in interstitial disease of the lungs. Amer. J. Med., *27*: 545-550, 1959.
100. Forster, R. E., Craw, M. R., Constantine, H. P., and Morello, J. A.: Gas exchange processes in the pulmonary capillaries. In: de Reuck, A. V. S., and O'Connor, M. (eds.), Ciba Foundation: Symposium on Pulmonary Structure and Function. London, J. & A. Churchill, 1962, pp. 215-231.
101. Milic-Emili, J., Henderson, J. A. M., Dolovich, M. B., Trop, D., and Kaneko, K.: Regional distribution of inspired gas in the lung. I. J. Appl. Physiol., *21*:749-759, 1966.
102. Ball, W. C., Jr., Stewart, P. B., Newsham, L. G. S., and Bates, D. V.: Regional pulmonary function studied with Xenon^{133}. J. Clin. Invest., *41*: 519-531, 1962.
103. West, J. B., and Dollery, C. T.: Distribution of blood flow and ventilation-perfusion ratio in the lung, measured with radioactive CO_2. J. Appl. Physiol., *15*:405-410, 1960.
104. Glazier, Jon B., and DeNardo, G. L.: Pulmonary function studied with the Xenon^{133} scanning technique. Normal values and a postural study. Amer. Rev. Resp. Dis., *94*:188-194, 1966.
105. Bentwoglio, L. G., Beerel, F., Stewart, P. B., Bryan, A. C., Ball, W. C., Jr., and Bates, D. V.: Studies of regional ventilation and perfusion in pulmonary emphysema using Xenon^{133}. Amer. Rev. Resp. Dis., *88*:315-329, 1963.
106. West, J. B., Dollery, C. T., and Hugh-Jones, P.: The use of radioactive carbon dioxide to measure regional blood flow in the lungs of patients with pulmonary disease. J. Clin. Invest., *40*:1-12, 1961.

107. West, J. B.: Ventilation/Blood Flow and Gas Exchange. Oxford, Blackwell, 1965.
108. Butler, J., and Somers, K.: Surface tension and the pericapillary pressure in the lungs. Fed. Proc. 22: (Abstr. 1071), 339, 1963.
109. Lloyd, Thomas C., Jr., and Wright, G. W.: Pulmonary vascular resistance and vascular transmural gradient. J. Appl. Physiol., *15*:241-245, 1960.
110. Hampton, C. S., and Chaloner, A.: Which stethoscope? Brit. Med. J., *4*:388-390, 1967.
111. Holley, H. S., Milic-Emili, J., Becklake, M. R., and Bates, D. V.: Regional distribution of pulmonary ventilation and perfusion in obesity. J. Clin. Invest., *46*:475-481, 1967.
112. Trapnell, David H.: Recognition and incidence of intrapulmonary lymph nodes. Thorax, *19*: 44-50, 1964.
113. Greenberg, Harry B.: Benign subpleural lymph node appearing as a pulmonary "coin" lesion. Radiology, *77*:97-99, 1961.
114. Rouvière, H.: Anatomy of the Human Lymphatic System. (Translated by Tobias, M. J.) Ann Arbor, Mich., Edwards, 1938.
115. McCort, James J., and Robbins, L. L.: Roentgen diagnosis of intrathoracic lymph-node metastases in carcinoma of the lung. Radiology, *57*:339-360, 1951.
116. Nohl, H. C.: An investigation into the lymphatic and vascular spread of carcinoma of the bronchus. Thorax, *11*:172-185, 1956.
117. Klingenberg, Inge: Histopathologic findings in the prescalene tissue from 1,000 post-mortem cases. Acta Chir. Scand., *127*:57-66, 1964.
118. Baird, James A.: The pathways of lymphatic spread of carcinoma of the lung. Brit. J. Surg., *52*:868-875, 1965.
119. Felson, Benjamin: The lobes and interlobar pleura: fundamental roentgen considerations. Amer. J. Med. Sci., *230*:572-584, 1955.
120. Kerley, P.: In: Shanks, S. C., and Kerley, P. (eds.), A Textbook of X-ray Diagnosis, Vol II (3rd ed.). Philadelphia, W. B. Saunders, 1962, p. 403.
121. Ritter, H., and Eyband, M.: Der diagnostische Werteines lageveränderten Ober-Mittellappenspaltes in Lungensagittalbild. (The diagnostic significance, in the sagittal chest film, of a shift in the upper and middle lobe fissures.) Fortschr. Roentgenst., *86*:431-439, 1957.
122. Simon, George: Principles of Chest X-ray Diagnosis. Philadelphia, F. A. Davis, 1956.
123. Schaffner: Chest. In: Shanks, S. C., and Kerley, P. (eds.), A Textbook of X-ray Diagnosis, Vol II (2nd ed.). Philadelphia, W. B. Saunders, 1950-1952, p. 241.
124. Simon, G.: Personal communication, 1967.
125. Boyden, Edward A.: Cleft left upper lobes and the split anterior bronchus. Surgery, *26*:167-180, 1949.
126. Davis, L. A.: The vertical fissure line. Amer. J. Roentgen., *84*:451-453, 1960.
127. Webber, Milo M., and O'Loughlin, B. J.: Variations of the pleural vertical fissure line. Radiology, *82*:461-462, 1964.
128. Friedman, Eliezer: Further observations on the vertical fissure line. Amer. J. Roentgen., *97*:171-173, 1966.
129. Rutishauser, Wilhelm J., Banchero, Natalio, Tsakiris, Amastasios G., Edmundowicz, Alphonse C., and Wood, Earl H.: Pleural pressures at dorsal and ventral sites in supine and prone body positions. J. Appl. Physiol., *21*:1500-1510, 1966.
130. Agostoni, E., and Mead, J.: Statics of the respiratory system. In: Fenn, W. O., and Rahn, H. (eds.), Handbook of Physiology. Section 3, Respiration. Vol. 1. Washington, American Physiological Society, 1964, p. 387-409.
131. Agostoni, E., Taglietti, A., and Setnikar, I.: Absorption force of the capillaries of the visceral pleura in determination of the intrapleural pressure. Amer. J. Physiol., *191*:277-282, 1957.
132. Brailsford, James F.: The radiographic posteromedial border of the lung, or the linear thoracic paraspinal shadow. Radiology, *41*:34-37, 1943.
133. Dalton, Catherine J., and Schwartz, S. S.: Evaluation of the paraspinal line in roentgen examination of the thorax. Radiology, *66*:195-200, 1956.
134. Cimmino, Christian V.: The anterior mediastinal line on chest roentgenograms. Radiology, *82*: 459-460, 1964.
135. Cimmino, Christian V., and Snead, L. O., Jr.: The posterior mediastinal line on chest roentgenograms. Radiology, *84*:516-518, 1965.
136. Cimmino, Christian V.: The esophageal-pleural stripe on chest teleroentgenograms. Radiology, *67*:754-756, 1956.
137. Cimmino, Christian V.: Further notes on the esophageal-pleural stripe. Radiology, *77*:974-978, 1961.
138. Ormond, Robert S., Jaconette, J. R., and Templeton, A. W.: The pleural esophageal reflection: an aid in the evaluation of esophageal disease. Radiology, *80*:738-742, 1963.
139. Lodin, H.: Mediastinal herniation and displacement studied by transversal tomography. Acta Radiol., *48*:337-350, 1957.
140. Gondos, B.: The roentgen image of the subclavian artery in the pulmonary apex. Amer. J. Roentgen., *86*:1058-1062, 1961.
141. Fleischner, F. G., and Udis, S. W.: Dilatation of the azygos veins: a roentgen sign of venous engorgement. Amer. J. Roentgen., *67*:569-575, 1952.
142. Doyle, F. H., Read, A. E., and Evans, K. T.: The mediastinum in portal hypertension. Clin. Radiol., *12*:114-129, 1961.
143. Lennon, E. A., and Simon, G.: The height of the diaphragm in the chest radiograph of normal adults. Brit. J. Radiol., *38*:937-943, 1965.
144. Wittenborg, M. H., and Aviad, I.: Organ influence on the normal posture of the diaphragm: a radiological study of inversions and heterotaxies. Brit. J. Radiol., *36*:280-288, 1963.
145. Köhler, Alban: Borderlands of the Normal and Early Pathologic in Skeletal Roentgenology (10th ed.). New York, Grune and Stratton, 1956.
146. Scheff, Saul, and Laforet, E. G.: The internal thoracic muscle and the lateral chest roentgenogram. Radiology, *86*:27-30, 1966.
147. Weinstein, Aaron S., and Mueller, C. F.: Intrathoracic rib. Amer. J. Roentgen., *94*:587-590, 1965.
148. Dunnill, M. S.: Postnatal growth of the lung. Thorax, *17*:329-333, 1962.
149. Loyd, Herbert M., String, S. T., and DuBois, A. B.: Radiographic and plethysmographic deter-

mination of total lung capacity. Radiology, *86*: 7-14, 1966.
150. Sackner, Marvin A., Feisal, K. A., and DuBois, A. B.: Determination of tissue volume and carbon dioxide dissociation slope of the lungs in man. J. Appl. Physiol., *19*:374-380, 1964.
151. McGaff, Charles J., Roveti, G. C., Glassman, E., and Milnor, W. R.: The pulmonary blood volume in rheumatic heart disease and its alteration by isoproterenol. Circulation, *27*:77-84, 1963.
152. Goldman, H. I., and Becklake, M. R.: Respiratory function tests: normal values at median altitudes and the prediction of normal results. Amer. Rev. Tuberc., *79*:457-467, 1959.
153. Newhouse, Michael T., Becklake, Margaret R., Macklem, Peter T., and McGregor, Maurice: Effect of alterations in end-tidal CO_2 tension on flow resistance. J. App. Physiol., *19*:745-749, 1964.
154. Flatley, F. Joseph, Constantine, H., McCredie, R. M., and Yu, P. N.: Pulmonary diffusing capacity and pulmonary capillary blood volume in normal subjects and in cardiac patients. Amer. Heart J., *64*:159-168, 1962.
155. Bucci, Giovanni, and Cook, C. D.: Studies on respiratory physiology in children. VI. Lung diffusing capacity, diffusing capacity of the pulmonary membrane and pulmonary capillary blood volume in congenital heart disease. J. Clin. Invest., *40*:1431-1441, 1961.
156. Jonsson, B., Linderholm, H., and Pinardi, G.: Atrial septal defect: a study of physical working capacity and hemodynamics during exercise. Acta Med. Scand., *159*:275-294, 1957.
157. Westermark, Nils: On the roentgen diagnosis of lung embolism. Acta Radiol., *19*:357-372, 1938.
158. Reid, Lynne, and Simon, G.: The peripheral pattern in the normal bronchogram and its relation to peripheral pulmonary anatomy. Thorax, *13*: 103-109, 1958.
159. Lavender, J. P., and Doppman, J.: The hilum in pulmonary venous hypertension. Brit. J. Radiol., *35*:303-313, 1962.
160. Daley, R., Goodwin, J. F., and Steiner, R. E. (eds.): Clinical Disorders of the Pulmonary Circulation. London, J. & A. Churchill, 1960.
161. Simon, G.: Personal communication, 1967.
162. Simon, G.: Personal communication, 1965.
163. Dollery, C. T., West, J. B., Wilcken, D. E. L., and Hugh-Jones, P.: A comparison of the pulmonary blood flow between left and right lungs in normal subjects and patients with congenital heart disease. Circulation, *24*:617-625, 1961.
164. Riley, R. L.: Effect of lung inflation upon the pulmonary vascular bed. In: de Reuck, A. V. S., and O'Connor, M. (eds.), Ciba Foundation: Symposium on Pulmonary Structure and Function. London, J. & A. Churchill, 1962, pp. 261-272.
165. Rigler, L. G.: Functional roentgen diagnosis: anatomical image – physiological interpretation. Amer. J. Roentgen., *82*:1-24, 1959.
166. Whitley, Joseph E., and Martin, J. F.: The Valsalva maneuver in roentgenologic diagnosis. Amer. J. Roentgen., *91*:297-306, 1964.
167. Westermark, Nils: On the influence of the intraalveolar pressure on the normal and pathological structure of the lungs. Acta Radiol., *25*:874-882, 1944.
168. Amundsen, Per: Planigraphy in Möller and Valsalva experiments. Acta Radiol., *40*:387-394, 1953.
169. Gamsu, Gordon, Thurlbeck, W. M., Macklem, P. T., and Fraser, R. G.: Peripheral bronchographic morphology in the normal human lung. In process of publication.
170. Gamsu, Gordon, Thurlbeck, W: M., Macklem, P. T., and Fraser, R. G.: The roentgenologic appearance of the human pulmonary acinus. In process of publication.
171. Jameson, A. Gregory: Diffusion of gases from alveolus to precapillary arteries. Science, *139*: 826-828, 1963.
172. Collier, Clarence R.: Determination of mixed venous CO_2 tensions by rebreathing. J. Appl. Physiol., *9*:25-29, 1956.
173. Campbell, E. J. M., and Howell, J. B. L.: Rebreathing method for measurement of mixed venous P_{CO_2}. Brit. Med. J., *2*:630–633, 1962.
174. Bates, D. V., Woolf, C. R., and Paul, G. I.: Chronic bronchitis: A report on the first two stages of the co-ordinated study of chronic bronchitis in the Department of Veterans Affairs, Canada. Med. Ser. J. Canad., *18*:211-303, 1962.
175. Trapnell, David H.: The peripheral lymphatics of the lung. Brit. J. Radiol., *36*:660–672, 1963.
176. Stewart, P. B.: The rate of formation and lymphatic removal of fluid in pleural effusions. J. Clin. Invest., *42*:258–262, 1963.
177. Stewart, P. B.: Personal communication, 1967.
178. Courtice, F. C., and Simmonds, W. J.: Absorption from the lungs. J. Physiol., *109*:103–116, 1949.
179. Nordenström, B., Effat, H., and Wojtowicz, J.: The use of elevated intrabronchial pressure for the demonstration of anomalous pulmonary veins and atrial defects. Brit. J. Radiol., *38*:762–765, 1965.
180. Burgen, A. S. V., and Stewart, P. B.: A method for measuring the turnover of fluid in the pleural and other serous cavities. J. Laborat. Clin. Med., *52*:118–124, 1958.
181. Boyden, Edward A.: The distribution of bronchi in gross anomalies of the right upper lobe, particularly lobes subdivided by the azygos vein and those containing pre-eparterial bronchi. Radiology, *58*:797–807, 1952.
182. Felson, Benjamin: Letter from the editor. Seminars in Roentgenol., *2*:323-324, 1967.
183. Keats, Theodore E., Lipscomb, G. E., and Betts, C. S., III: Mensuration of the arch of the azygos vein and its application to the study of cardiopulmonary disease. Radiology, *90*:990-994, 1968.
184. Goldenberg, David B., and Brogdon, B. G.: Congenital anomalies of the pectoral girdle demonstrated by chest radiography. J. Canad. Ass. Radiol., *18*:472-477, 1967.
185. Parsons, F. G.: On the proportions and characteristics of the modern English clavicle. J. Anat., *51*:71-93, 1917.
186. Shauffer, Irving A., and Collins, W. V.: The deep clavicular rhomboid fossa. Clinical significance and incidence in 10,000 routine chest photofluorograms. J.A.M.A., *195*:778-779, 1966.
187. Shopfner, Chas. E., Jansen, C., and O'Kell, R. T.: Roentgen significance of the transverse thoracis muscle. Amer. J. Roentgen., *103*:140-148, 1968.
188. Sanders, C. F.: Sexing by costal cartilage calcification, Brit. J. Radiol., *39*:233, 1966.
189. Holland, J., Milic-Emili, J., Macklem, P. T., and

Bates, D. V.: Regional distribution of pulmonary ventilation and perfusion in elderly subjects. J. Clin. Invest., *47*:81-92, 1968.

190. Anthonisen, N. R., Bass, H., and Heckscher, T.: ^{133}Xe Studies of patients after pneumonectomy. Scand. J. Resp. Dis., *49*:81-91, 1968.

191. Bass, H., Heckscher, T., and Anthonisen, N. R.: Regional pulmonary gas exchange in patients with pulmonary embolism. Clin. Sci., *33*:355-364, 1967.

192. Anthonisen, N. R., Bass, H., Heckscher, T., Oriol, A., and Bates, D. V.: Recent observation on the measurement of regional V/Q ratios in chronic lung disease. J. Nucl. Biol. Med., *11*:73-79, 1967.

193. Anthonisen, N. R., Dolovich, M. B., and Bates, D. V.: Steady state measurement of regional ventilation to perfusion ratios in normal man. J. Clin. Invest., *45*:1349-1356, 1966.

194. Bryan, A. C., Bentivoglio, L. G., Beerel, F., MacLeish, H., Zidulka, A., and Bates, D. V.: Factors affecting regional distribution of ventilation and perfusion in the lung. J. Appl. Physiol., *19*:395-402, 1964.

195. Barnhard, Howard J., Pierce, J. A., Joyce, J. W., and Bates, J. H.: Roentgenographic determination of total lung capacity. A new method evaluated in health, emphysema and congestive heart failure. Amer. J. Med., *28*:51–60, 1960.

196. Nicklaus, Ted M., Watanabe, S., Mitchell, M. M., and Renzetti, A. D., Jr.: Roentgenologic, physiologic and structural estimations of the total lung capacity in normal and emphysematous subjects. Amer. J. Med., *42*:547-553, 1967.

197. Stamm, Stanley J.: Reliability of capillary blood for the measurement of pO_2 and O_2 saturation. Dis. Chest, *52*:191-194, 1967.

198. Gorlin, R., Lewis, B. M., Haynes, F. W., Spiegl, R. J., and Dexter, L.: Factors regulating pulmonary "capillary" pressure in mitral stenosis. Amer. Heart J., *41*:834-854, 1951.

199. Georg, J., Lassen, N. A., Millemgaard, K., and Vinther, A.: Diffusion in the gas phase of the lungs in normal and emphysematous subjects. Clin. Sci., *29*:525–532, 1965.

200. Webb, Watts R., Lanius, J. W., Aslami, A., and Reynold, R. C.: The effects of hyperbaric-oxygen tensions on pulmonary surfactant in guinea pigs and rats. J.A.M.A., *195*:279-280, 1966.

201. Macklem, Peter T., and Mead, J.: Resistance of central and peripheral airways measured by a retrograde catheter. J. Appl. Physiol., *22*:395-401, 1967.

202. Piiper, Johannes, Haab, P., and Rahn, H.: Unequal distribution of pulmonary diffusing capacity in the anesthetized dog. J. Appl. Physiol., *16*:499-506, 1961.

INDEX

Note: Page numbers in *italics* indicate illustrations; (t) indicates table.